PACIFIC SOCIAL WORK

As a region, the Pacific is changing rapidly. This edited collection, the first of its kind, centres Pacific-Indigenous ways of knowing, doing and being in Pacific social work. In so doing, the authors decolonise the dominant western rhetoric that is evident in contemporary social work practice in the region and rejuvenate practice models with evolving Pacific perspectives. *Pacific Social Work*:

- Incorporates Pacific epistemologies and ontologies in social and community work practice, social policy and research
- Profiles contemporary Pacific needs – including health, education, environmental, justice and welfare
- Demonstrates the application of Pacific-Indigenous knowledges in practice in diverse Pacific contexts
- Examines Pacific-Indigenous research approaches to promote inform practice and positive outcomes
- Reviews Pacific models of social and community work and their application
- Fosters Pacific perspectives for social work and community work education and training in the Pacific region

Pacific Social Work demonstrates the role of social work within societies where social and cultural differences are evident, and practitioners, community groups, researchers, educators and governments are encouraged to consider the integration between local indigenous and international knowledge and practice. Providing rigorously researched case studies, questions and exercises, this book will be a key learning resource for social work and human and community services students, practitioners, social services managers and policy makers in Australia, New Zealand and various Pacific Island states across the Pacific, including Fiji, Tonga, Samoa, Vanuatu and Papua New Guinea.

Jioji Ravulo is an Associate Professor in Social Work at the University of Wollongong, Australia. His father is iTaukei Fijian and mother is Anglo-Australian. He is passionate about diversity and its differences, and how this can be meaningfully included in the work being undertaken in Pacific social work across Oceania and alongside the Pacific diaspora globally.

Tracie Malfile'o is a Senior Lecturer in the School of Social Work, Massey University New Zealand. She is a second generation Pacific New Zealander; her late father Mohetau Sosaia Mafile'o hailed from Te'ekiu in Tonga and also had genealogy linking to Nukulaelae, Tuvalu. Her career has involved two decades in academic roles across New Zealand and Papua New Guinea focusing on Pacific culture-based scholarship, social development and social work.

Donald Bruce Yeates has held senior academic and administrative positions at the University of Papua New Guinea and The University of the South Pacific. He has lived in the Pacific for the last 44 years and is a Fijian/Canadian dual citizen. He is passionate about social and community work practice and its realisation of social and ecological justice in the Pacific and beyond.

PACIFIC SOCIAL WORK

Navigating Practice, Policy
and Research

*Edited by Jioji Ravulo, Tracie Mafile'o
and Donald Bruce Yeates*

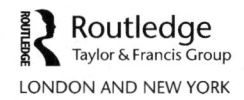

Routledge
Taylor & Francis Group
LONDON AND NEW YORK

First published 2019
by Routledge
2 Park Square, Milton Park, Abingdon, Oxon OX14 4RN

and by Routledge
711 Third Avenue, New York, NY 10017

Routledge is an imprint of the Taylor & Francis Group, an informa business

© 2019 selection and editorial matter, Jioji Ravulo, Tracie Mafile'o and Donald Bruce Yeates; individual chapters, the contributors

The right of Jioji Ravulo, Tracie Mafile'o and Donald Bruce Yeates to be identified as the authors of the editorial material, and of the authors for their individual chapters, has been asserted in accordance with sections 77 and 78 of the Copyright, Designs and Patents Act 1988.

All rights reserved. No part of this book may be reprinted or reproduced or utilised in any form or by any electronic, mechanical, or other means, now known or hereafter invented, including photocopying and recording, or in any information storage or retrieval system, without permission in writing from the publishers.

Trademark notice: Product or corporate names may be trademarks or registered trademarks, and are used only for identification and explanation without intent to infringe.

British Library Cataloguing-in-Publication Data
A catalogue record for this book is available from the British Library

Library of Congress Cataloging-in-Publication Data
Names: Ravulo, Jioji, author. | Mafile'o, Tracie, author. | Yeates, Donald Bruce, author.
Title: Pacific social work: navigating practice, policy and research/ Jioji Ravulo, Tracie Malfile'o and Donald Bruce Yeates.
Description: 1st Edition. | New York: Routledge, 2019. | Includes bibliographical references and index.
Identifiers: LCCN 2018055137 | ISBN 9781138501300 (hardback) | ISBN 9781138501317 (pbk.) | ISBN 9781315144252 (ebook)
Subjects: LCSH: Social service—Pacific Area. | Pacific Area—Social policy. | Social service—Research.
Classification: LCC HV405.3 .R38 2019 | DDC 361.30995–dc23
LC record available at https://lccn.loc.gov/2018055137

ISBN: 978-1-138-50130-0 (hbk)
ISBN: 978-1-138-50131-7 (pbk)
ISBN: 978-1-315-14425-2 (ebk)

Typeset in Bembo
by Deanta Global Publishing Services, Chennai, India

CONTENTS

List of figures — viii
List of tables — ix
List of contributors — x
Foreword by James Midgley — xv
Acknowledgements — xix

PART I
Pacific social work — 1

1 Introduction to Pacific social work: Places, peoples, perspectives and practices — 3
  Jioji Ravulo, Tracie Mafile'o and Donald Bruce Yeates

2 Contemporary Pacific values and beliefs — 11
  Aliitasi Su'a-Tavila

3 Pacific-Indigenous social work theories and models — 22
  Tracie Mafile'o, Jean Mitaera and Karlo Mila

PART II
Fields of practice — 35

4 Seeing abilities: Disability in the Pacific — 37
  Donald Bruce Yeates

5   Understanding mental health and wellbeing from
    a Pacific perspective   47
    Jioji Ravulo, Monique Faleafa and Tanya Koro

6   Environmental justice and social work in climate change
    in the Pacific Islands   58
    Dora Kuir-Ayius and David Marena

7   Pacific-Indigenous community-village resilience in disasters   68
    Siautu Alefaio-Tugia, Emeline Afeaki-Mafile'o and Petra Satele

8   Delivering youth justice for Pacific young people
    and their families   79
    Jioji Ravulo, Jack Scanlan and Vivian Koster

9   Applying culturally appropriate approaches when working
    with Pacific adult offenders   90
    Jioji Ravulo and Julia Ioane

10 Community development: Connecting research, policy and
    practice in Pacific communities   102
    Dunstan Lawihin, Wheturangi Walsh-Tapiata and Kesaia Vasutoga

11 Understanding the Vā for social work engagement with
    Pacific women and children   114
    Selina Ledoux-Taua'aletoa

12 An introduction to sexual and reproductive health and
    wellbeing for Pacific social work   125
    Michelle Redman-MacLaren and Analosa Veukiso-Ulugia

13 Getting on the K.A.D.: The impacts of kava, alcohol and
    other drug consumption across Pacific communities   139
    Moses Ma'alo Faleolo and Jioji Ravulo

14 Our Pacific elders as keepers and transmitters of culture   150
    Halaevalu F. Ofahengaue Vakalahi and Ofa K.L. Hafoka-Kanuch

15 Understanding sexual and gender diversity in
    the Pacific Islands   161
    Geir Henning Presterudstuen

16 Family and domestic violence   172
    Yvonne Crichton-Hill and Rebecca Olul

17 Global migration and resettlement: A case study on
    the Fijian experience   184
    Litea Meo-Sewabu

PART III
Social policy   **195**

18 Navigating social policy processes in the Pacific   197
    Leituala Kuiniselani Toelupe Tago-Elisara and Donald Bruce Yeates

PART IV
Research   **207**

19 Towards a Pacific-Indigenous research paradigm for
    Pacific social work   209
    Tracie Mafile'o, Peter Mataira and Kate Saxton

PART V
Future directions   **221**

20 Where to from here?: Integration of indigenous knowledges
    and practice in contemporary settings   223
    Jioji Ravulo and Wheturangi Walsh-Tapiata

Index   *233*

FIGURES

3.1	Mapping of Pacific social work theories and models	25
3.2	The continuum of wellbeing	26
7.1	Pacific-Indigenous disaster response	72
7.2	Vision of Talanoa HUBBS hosted in Tonga by Tupu'anga Café	75
7.3	2017 Delegates in full talanoa-mode (Author)	75
7.4	2018 Talanoa HUBBS in Tonga hosted by Tupu'anga Café (Author)	77
18.1	Social policy process in the Pacific	200

TABLES

1.1	Terms to describe Pacific people	7
2.1	Glossary of Samoan terms used within chapter	20
6.1	Climate change policy frameworks and programmes for PICs	59
8.1	Pacific youth risk & protective factors	83
9.1	Promoting restorative justice with adults across Pacific social work	96
12.1	Interrelated features required to experience positive sexual health	128
12.2	Examples of international, regional and national policy organisations	134
15.1	Glossary of terms used within Chapter	169
17.1	Glossary of terms used within Chapter	191
19.1	Pacific-Indigenous research paradigm: Ontology, epistemology, axiology and methodology	213

CONTRIBUTORS

Emeline Afeaki-Mafile'o is a PhD Candidate with the School of Psychology at Massey University, Auckland, New Zealand. Her father is Tongan, Samoan and Maori and her mother is Tongan and Samoan. She founded Affirming Works in 2001, which uses a Pacific model of collective mentoring to provide mentoring and educational life skills to young people, their families and communities. She is a social entrepreneur who embraces her diverse ethnicities whilst using her eclectic skills of social work, social policy and business to address issues of poverty in our Pacific communities.

Siautu Alefaio-Tugia is a Senior Lecturer at the School of Psychology at Massey University, Auckland, New Zealand and has a Samoan lineage from the villages of Matautu-Tai, Sasina and Manunu ma Fagamalo. She is an experienced psychologist practitioner that has worked across various applied psychology contexts in education, health, social services, community, family violence, forensic rehabilitation and disaster humanitarian response in Aotearoa New Zealand, Australia and the Pacific. As a pracademic, she combines extensive practice and academic experience to re-inform psychology from Pacific-Indigenous knowledge frameworks.

Yvonne Crichton-Hill is a Senior Lecturer in the social work programme at the University of Canterbury, New Zealand. Her father is Samoan and her mother is of English and Australian descent. Yvonne is passionate about working with Pasifika people and communities to grow both community and policy responses that enhance the lives of Pasifika people.

Monique Faleafa is a registered clinical psychologist and has served her Pacific communities in the not-for-profit sector, district health boards, academia and social services for over 20 years as a clinician and as an advocate for improving equity in health and social outcomes for Pacific and disadvantaged communities. Monique is

Contributors xi

the founding Chief Executive of Le Va, a national non-government organisation (NGO) in New Zealand focused on Pacific people's wellbeing. She also contributes to her communities at governance levels, serving on crown entities, science and research boards and regulatory authorities.

Moses Ma'alo Faleolo is an Academic from Massey University, Auckland, New Zealand. He is a New Zealand-born Samoan and holds a paramount chiefly title, Gisa from Falelima, Samoa. His father, Leaula, and late mother, Pepe, is where he draws his passion and knowledge from including how Pacific concepts can be applied in social work education, practice and policy development.

Ofa K.L. Hafoka-Kanuch is a graduate with a PhD in Counseling Psychology from the APA-accredited programme at Brigham Young University, Utah, the Unites States. She completed an APA-accredited predoctoral internship at the Brigham Young University Counseling and Psychological Services. She is passionate about helping people love fully, live authentically and find meaning, healing and balance in their lives.

Julia Ioane is a lecturer in Psychology at the Auckland University of Technology (AUT), Aotearoa New Zealand and a clinical psychologist in private practice within the Justice sector. She is Samoan from the villages of Fasito'outa and Leauva'a in Samoa. Julia is passionate about including Pasifika worldviews, epistemology and practice within the realm of psychology and promoting Pasifika understanding in working among Pasifika people with offending behaviour.

Tanya Koro is the co-founder of Amanaki STEM Academy, fostering Pacific student success in the sciences. She is a proud Tokelauan/Samoan and lives in New Zealand with her husband and three children. She is fluent in her languages and cultures thanks to her upbringing in Samoa surrounded by her Tokelauan families. Tanya has worked as a Psychiatric Social Worker and Pasifika Mental Health Clinical Consult Liaison for MidCentral District Health Board in New Zealand. She is passionate about community development with a focus on enhancing protective factors for Pasifika youth and their families.

Vivian Koster is a PhD student in the Faculty of Arts, Law and Education, School of Social Sciences at the University of the South Pacific, Suva, Fiji.

Dora Kuir-Ayius is a Lecturer in Social Work at the University of Papua New Guinea, Port Moresby, Papua New Guinea. She is a Melanesian who is passionate about building community resilience in mining communities as well as other development issues including those in social work within and beyond the Pacific.

Dunstan Lawihin is a Tutor in Social Work at the University of Papua New Guinea, Port Moresby, Papua New Guinea. His parents are both natural indigenous Papua

New Guineans living a traditional subsistence life. He is passionate about developing culturally relevant social work education by connecting the local and global commonalities and differences in order to appreciate the uniqueness of social work education and practice in the Pacific and across the globe.

Selina Ledoux-Taua'aletoa is a Lecturer and Academic Leader in Social Practice at Unitec, Auckland, New Zealand.

Tracie Mafile'o is a Senior Lecturer in the School of Social Work, Massey University, New Zealand. She is a second generation Pacific New Zealander, her late father Mohetau Sosaia Mafile'o hailed from Te'ekiu in Tonga and also had genealogy linking to Nukulaelae, Tuvalu. Her career has involved two decades in academic roles across New Zealand and Papua New Guinea, focusing on Pacific culture-based scholarship, social development and social work.

David Marena is the Chief Executive Officer of Mortlock (Takuu) Island Climate Change Association (MICCA) and is based in Buka, Autonomous Region of Bougainville, Papua New Guinea.

Peter Mataira is an Associate Professor in Social Work at Hawai'i Pacific University on Oahu, Hawai', the United States. He is Maori of Ngatiporou, Te Aitanga-a-Mahaki and Kahungunu descent and is passionate about Indigenous human and economic rights, social and environmental justice, research and (re)empowerment. He teaches community practice, social entrepreneurship, human behaviour in the social environment and sustainability.

Litea Meo-Sewabu is a Lecturer in Social Work and Social Policy, and Programme Coordinator of Social Work in the School of Social Sciences, Faculty of Arts, Law and Education at the University of the South Pacific, Suva, Fiji.

Karlo Mila is a Poet and Academic with heritage from Tonga, Samoa and Europe. She is an acclaimed author and writer, with specific focus on Pacific people and their identities. She has worked extensively in many fields, including mental health, wellbeing, Pacific models and theories.

Jean Mitaera is the Chief Advisor of Pacific Strategy at Wellington Institute of Technology & Whitireia Community Polytechnic, Wellington, New Zealand. She is Cook Islands Maori and taught social work for 26 years. She was the lead writer of Turanga Māori and a facilitator of the Pacific family violence training programme. Jean enjoys conversations that explore Pacific epistemologies, frameworks and models of research and practice.

Rebecca Olul is the Communications Officer at the UNICEF Vanuatu Field Office in Port Vila, Vanuatu. She is of ni-Vanuatu heritage; her father comes from the island of Pentecost and mother from Tanna in the south. She is passionate about working to make a change in the lives of children, youth and women in Vanuatu and the greater Pacific.

Geir Henning Presterudstuen is a Lecturer in Anthropology at Western Sydney University, Australia. He has conducted ethnographic fieldwork in urban Fiji since 2009 where he works with socially and culturally diverse communities to promote social justice and Pacific forms of knowledge as integral to social analysis.

Jioji Ravulo is an Associate Professor in Social Work at the University of Wollongong, Australia. His father is iTaukei Fijian and mother is Anglo Australian. He is passionate about diversity and its differences, and how this can be meaningfully included in the work being undertaken in Pacific social work across Oceania and alongside the Pacific diaspora globally.

Michelle Redman-MacLaren is a Senior Research Fellow at James Cook University, Australia. Redman-MacLaren, who has Anglo-Celtic ancestry, has worked with Pacific and Indigenous Australian communities for more than two decades. She is passionate about facilitating and supporting action-oriented research in a culturally respectful way for positive health and social outcomes.

Petra Satele is part of New IndigenoUs Unity of Pacific Humanitarians (NIUPacH), a Pacific research collective based at Massey University, New Zealand, where she is continuing her studies in humanitarian and indigenous psychology. She is of Samoan descent and has studied psychology at Brigham Young University Hawaii, the United States.

Kate Saxton is a Social Work Lecturer at Australian Catholic University in Brisbane, Australia. She has previously lived in Fiji and Tonga where she both taught and worked as a social work practitioner before returning to Australia to be closer to her family. Kate has a strong interest in Indigenous research methodologies and culturally responsive approaches to research design and implementation. She is committed to promoting decolonising approaches to social work in both practice, research and teaching.

Jack Scanlan is currently completing a Doctor of Social Work degree at Massey University. He is a New Zealand-born Samoan and his late parents were from the villages of Faleula and Vaiusu/Vaigaga. He holds a Bachelors of Arts degree majoring in Sociology and a Master of Social Work applied degree with honours. His research focus is on Pasifika, specifically Samoan youth offending, which stems from over 20 years' experience in the youth justice field. Jack is happily married to his wife Nicky, who is of Ngati Tuwharetoa/Māori descent, and they have three children.

Aliitasi Su'a-Tavila is a Programme Manager, Professional Practice at Whitireia and WelTec Institutions, Wellington, New Zealand. She is a Samoan woman who is passionate about blending Pacific cultural values and beliefs to social work practice to ensure it manifested across the Pacific diaspora.

Leituala Kuiniselani Toelupe Tago-Elisara is a Samoan national and currently the Director for the Social Development Programme at the Pacific Community (SPC) in Suva, Fiji. She is passionate about serving and helping Pacific people advance their goals and aspirations and utilising Pacific social work as a means to address challenges faced by families and communities.

Halaevalu F. Ofahengaue Vakalahi is the Dean of the College of Health and Society, School of Social Work at Hawai'i Pacific University, the United States.

Kesaia Vasutoga is a Teaching Assistant and Field Work Practice Educator at the University of the South Pacific, Laucala Campus, Suva, Fiji. She is of iTaukei Fijian descent, with both paternal and maternal links to Lau, a group of islands on the south eastern parts of Fiji that was once under the Tongan regime in the pre-colonial era. She is passionate about community development issues and how indigenous knowledge must be considered and included in the exchanges around developing communities in the Pacific.

Analosa Veukiso-Ulugia is a social work Lecturer at the University of Auckland, New Zealand, and is of Samoan descent. With extensive experience across clinical, research, management and community settings, her research focuses on Pacific sexual health and adolescent wellbeing. She is also exploring mechanisms that can enhance the success of Pacific students in tertiary education.

Wheturangi Walsh-Tapiata is the Chief Executive Officer of Te Oranganui Trust, a tribally led Health and Social Services NGO, where she works in the community. She has a Masters in Social Work from Massey University, Auckland, New Zealand. She has an extensive academic career, having worked at Massey University and Te Wānanga o Aotearoa, Aotearoa New Zealand. Her particular passions are teaching, research and practice that centres around indigenous social work and community development.

Donald Bruce Yeates has held senior academic and administrative positions at the University of Papua New Guinea and The University of the South Pacific. He has lived in the Pacific for the last 44 years and is a Fijian/Canadian dual citizen. He is passionate about social and community work practice and its realisation of social and ecological justice in the Pacific and beyond.

FOREWORD

Pacific social work: Navigating practice, policy and research

From its early beginnings in a handful of Western countries in the late 19th century, social work has emerged as an organised, global profession. Unlike the situation just a few decades ago when social work training was primarily offered in Western countries, professional social work training schools have been established all over the world, mostly at the university level. The International Association of Schools of Social Work now has more than 400 member schools in about 60 countries in all the world's regions. Employment opportunities for social workers have expanded not only in traditional social service agencies but in new and innovative fields of practice. Although the majority of social workers are engaged in conventional child welfare, mental health, medical social work and correctional programmes, they also work with poor rural communities, street children, refugees and trafficked women and children. Many are also involved in innovative development projects committed to meeting the United Nations' Sustainable Development Goals. Professional associations have been created in many countries to represent their members and often they lobby governments on issues related to social work practice. Today, the International Federation of Social Workers, which represents social work practitioners, has member associations in more than 80 countries. In addition, many governments have supported the profession by subsidising social work training and often regulations governing social work practice and the qualifications of social workers have been introduced.

The international expansion of the profession has been accompanied by a growing literature about social work education and practice in different parts of the world. Originally, academic studies of this kind were confined to Western countries but in recent times, much more information has become available about social work's multiple roles and functions in Africa, Asia, Oceania and Central and South America. In addition to providing historical and descriptive accounts of the profession's evolution and current activities, these studies address the numerous issues and challenges it faces around the world. Many also highlight its commitment to progressive social change and its efforts to promote social justice. A good deal of the literature has focused on social work's cultural relevance to the needs of diverse countries and the way social workers around the world are seeking to enhance its impact in the context of local realities. This reflects a growing commitment to decolonize social work and challenge the dominant Western narratives that have shaped the profession's global expansion. The critique of "professional imperialism" that I and other colleagues offered almost 40 years ago has helped to foster a greater awareness of the need for indigenisation and greater cultural relevance.

Although a great deal of progress has been made, it cannot be claimed that social work is always responsive to local needs and realities or that the profession has successfully met the challenges of practising effectively in diverse social and cultural contexts. Inappropriate practice methods adopted from Western countries continue to be employed and students from many countries continue to rely on textbooks imported from abroad that are of limited value in preparing them for practice in their own societies. In addition, social work all over the world is faced with overwhelming social need accompanied by a lack of resources as well as low professional status and limited public support. In some countries, entrenched negative attitudes towards those it serves impedes the profession's impact. In others, governments have adopted policies that have retrenched and curtailed the social services. Social work's ability to respond to new social needs has also been limited by insufficient resources and opportunities to implement innovative ideas.

Despite these challenges, there is little doubt that the global expansion of social work has been a remarkable development and that millions of people around the world have benefited from social work intervention. This should strengthen the resolve of social workers everywhere to continue the struggle to promote social wellbeing for all. This commitment will be fostered if social workers recognize that they are part of an international community of professionals who share common goals. In turn, this will be fostered by greater international exchanges between social workers from different parts of the world. As I have previously argued, social workers around the world have much to learn from each other. By sharing ideas and practice experiences, truly reciprocal learning can be fostered and international innovations can be adapted to meet local needs.

By documenting and discussing many of the issues the profession has addressed in the Pacific region, the editors and contributors to *Pacific Social Work: Navigating Practice, Policy and Research* make a major contribution to promoting positive international exchanges. Covering a vast territory comprised of mainly island nations, the region has not always been given proper attention by social workers in other parts of the world but, as the book reveals, its unique features and challenges will be of interest to social workers everywhere. Indeed, there is much to be learned from colleagues in the region who have adapted conventional practice methods and innovated with new ideas to respond to the issues facing its peoples. The book begins, by way of background, with three chapters that discuss the region's social, cultural, political, geographic, demographic and religious features which impinge on social work practice and require that social workers adopt indigenous perspectives that value the realities of the diverse member states that comprise the region. Recognising this diversity, the book's next chapter (Chapter 2) identifies the shared values and beliefs of the region's nations as well as the significant numbers living in the Pacific diaspora. The following and particularly important chapter (Chapter 3) discusses the different models of care and social development that have emerged to underpin culturally relevant practice in the region. These conceptual models have been adopted in different fields of practice and are highly instructive for social workers everywhere seeking to develop indigenous forms of practice.

The bulk of the book (Chapters 4 to 17) focus on the major fields of practice in which social workers in the region are engaged. These include familiar topics such as social work and mental health, disability, families and children, youth justice, elders, adult offending, alcohol and other drugs and domestic and family violence. In addition, a number of issues that are not always regarded as a part of mainstream social work are covered. They include sexual health and family planning, LGBTQI+ issues, migration and resettlement and disaster management and relief. Recognising the importance of the region's commitment to attain the Sustainable Development Goals, a useful chapter (Chapter 10) discusses community development and educational engagement designed to build community capacity and enhance the region's collectivist traditions. Another important chapter (Chapter 6) discusses climate change and the impact of global warming on the region's island low-lying countries. This issue has particular significance for the region but a greater global commitment to address the problem is also needed.

The book concludes with two chapters (Chapters 18 and 19) concerned with social policy and collaborative research as well as a final reflective chapter (Chapter 20) which speculates about future trends and the way social change will affect the region's peoples. Although globalisation, individualism and the adoption of market ideas will undoubtedly affect its traditional culture, the chapter urges social workers to understand these processes and maintain a critical lens which helps to navigate its future. It notes in particular that those living in the Pacific diaspora are especially exposed to new forces but urges social workers serving these clients to be attuned to their needs. As international migration accelerates, social workers everywhere need to be better informed about the cultures and backgrounds of their increasingly diverse communities they serve. Together with the growing literature on social work in different countries, this book will help them to understand the unique needs of these communities. Social work practitioners, social work researchers and educators should also consult this book. It offers valuable insights into social work's role and contribution in the region and it raises many interesting questions. Most helpfully, it shows how social workers will benefit from the experiences of their colleagues in this region of the world. I am honoured to write this Foreword to *Pacific Social Work* which is an important addition to the international social work literature. It deserves to be widely read.

James Midgley

ACKNOWLEDGEMENTS

We appreciate the various individuals that were involved in the collective effort of creating and establishing this edited collection; including our many authors from across Oceania and beyond who contributed to our 20 chapters, and James Midgley for his insightful Foreword. We are also grateful to those that assisted in the development and completion of this book including Laisani Petersen, Ipul Powesu, Kevin Dunn, Shannon Said and Chris Panagiotaros.

Thank you to the participants who came along to our initial writing workshop at the University of the South Pacific in March 2017 in Suva, Fiji: Viniana Cakau, Vilisi Gadolo, Lameka Koroi, Monika Koroi-Robinson, Titilia Lagilagi-Kedrabuka, David Merick, Tomasi Raiyawa, Leslie Tikotikoca, Joji Taqiritawa and Nanise Christine Waqamailau. We are also thankful for the support of Helen Simmons from Massey University for the Writing Retreat undertaken in September 2017 in Auckland, New Zealand.

We acknowledge the International Association of Schools of Social Work (IASSW) for their support of the Advancing Pacific Social Work Symposium held in Fiji, March 2017, and for instigating the newly formed Social Work Regional Resource Centre of Oceania (SWRROC).

We are also grateful for the institutions that provided support along the way: Massey University – School of Social Work, The University of the South Pacific – Faculty of Arts, Law and Education, School of Social Sciences, Western Sydney University – School of Social Sciences and Psychology and the University of Wollongong – Faculty of Social Sciences.

Overall, we are greatly humbled by the honour and privilege to put together a collection that strives to highlight the richness of our ancestral knowledges, values and beliefs. We are better as a collective due to our many Pacific Elders within our families and communities that continue to guide and lead our space and place within our Island homes, and the diaspora globally.

From the individual editors

Jioji Ravulo: Much appreciation Losana for all your support, guidance, inspiration, prayers, patience and shared vision in serving across the Pacific. To our son, Ratu Kini, continue to do you – we think you're amazing. To my parents, Jovesa Ravulo and the late Norelle Ravulo, thank you for always encouraging us to strive through education. And to my dear siblings, Kelera, Talei, Alana and Joey – thank you for your ongoing belief in what we do. And finally, to Tracie and Bruce – thanks for sharing this journey in exploring and navigating this exciting project. *Vinaka vaka levu.*

Tracie Mafile'o: My first acknowledgement goes to my late father Mohetau Sosaia Mafile'o who, during the writing of this book, passed away. His dedication to education and the wellbeing of future generations, rising out of the challenges within his own life journey, has been a key motivation in my scholarship. Secondly, thanks to my mother, Margaret Mafile'o, for extra school pick-ups and baby-sitting to free up my time. Finally, I acknowledge my husband Taupo Tani and my two young boys Tuviya and Timon, for bearing with me when I was not there because of projects such as this, and for focusing me on a future worth forging for Pacific families and communities. *'Ofa lahi atu.*

Donald Bruce Yeates: My heartfelt thank you to all friends, colleagues and former students of the Port Moresby Community Development Group, the University of Papua New Guinea and The University of the South Pacific. Your support of my social and community work journey in the Pacific through the last 44 years is greatly appreciated. A special thank you to Emeritus Professor Maev O'Collins who founded the Social Work Programme at the University of Papua New Guinea and mentored me through my early academic career. And to Jioji Ravulo and Tracie Mafile'o – thanks for letting me join you on this navigational adventure.

PART I
Pacific social work

1

INTRODUCTION TO PACIFIC SOCIAL WORK

Places, peoples, perspectives and practices

Jioji Ravulo, Tracie Mafile'o and Donald Bruce Yeates

Key points

- There are diverse ways in which the Pacific and its people are defined. Utilising appropriate and just language is important to promoting positive inclusion.
- The Pacific region has been subjected to many forms of social and economic development which should include culturally responsive social work.
- Utilising Pacific perspectives to inform practices is an important part of inclusion.
- A definition of Pacific social work operates from a desire to promote a shared and collective approach.

Introduction: The vision of Pacific social work

> The ocean ... is our most wonderful metaphor for just about anything we can think of. Contemplation of its vastness and majesty, its allurement and fickleness, its regularities and unpredictability, its shoals and depths, and its isolating and linking role in our histories, excites the imagination and kindles a sense of wonder, curiosity, and hope that could set us on journeys to explore new regions of creative enterprise that we have not dreamt of before.
>
> *(Hau'ofa, 1998, p. 406)*

Pacific social work holds a hopeful vision for the peoples and societies of the world's largest ocean and contributes an alternative vision for social work globally. The "Pacific" in Pacific social work recognises the utility of a regional identity based on our common inheritance of geographic, relational and cultural resources in Oceania (Hau'ofa, 1998). Pacific social work draws from ancient knowledges and ways which have persisted and adapted over time and space (Ka'ili, 2017; Mila, 2017). These Pacific-Indigenous knowledges and ways offer resources and strengths relevant for complexities and challenges facing Pacific communities.

We define Pacific social work as:

> *Centring Pacific-Indigenous ways of knowing and doing, being and becoming for community, family and individual wellbeing whilst counteracting structural, cultural and personal oppressions within Oceania and throughout the diaspora.*

In providing this definition, we are not wanting to limit the scope of Pacific social work, but instead create a platform for further *talanoa*, collaboration and development of the potential of Pacific social work to envision better conditions for ola/ora/wellbeing. We are promoting a collective approach where Pacific people are valued for their perspectives, for the lands and ocean from which they originate and for their activism as collaborators in change processes within various fields of practice.

In this book, *Pacific Social Work: Navigating Practice, Policy and Research*, contributors explore the application of Pacific perspectives in their respective fields of practice and the intersection of local, regional and international practice, policy and research. This chapter introduces the Pacific through a discussion of the places, peoples, perspectives and practices which constitute the context of Pacific social work.

Places and peoples

Pacific geo-politics is partly a treatise in oceanography.

> The environment of the small but vivacious communities of the islands is the nourishing, at times threatening, sea. Pacific Islander[s] ... have a special way of comprehending the world. ... Islanders live on small pieces of earth surrounded by the wealth – and menace – of the sea.
>
> *(Garrett, 1982, p. xi)*

Spanish, Dutch, British and French ships brought the explorers, scientists and Christian missionaries to the Pacific and were the genesis of colonisation. Within colonisation, the Pacific was sub-divided (rather inaccurately) into Melanesia, Micronesia and Polynesia. These sub-divisions are credited to the works of the French explorer Jules Dumont d'Urville. The divisions are drawn according to indigenous people's skin colour – mela (black) – and perceived types of islands – micro (small) and poly (many) (Lewis, 2018). These terms are still used in the geo-political language of today. The Melanesian Spearhead Group, the Polynesian Leaders' Group and the Micronesian Presidents' Group are all political sub-regional groups meeting to further the interests of those countries and territories in the areas of the Pacific in which they are situated.

Individual States and Non-Government Organisations (NGOs) are similarly grouped reflecting the structure of Pacific regionalism. Decisions and policies from these regional organisations are the manner in which the collective voice of the Pacific region is shaped and articulated in the global forums of the United Nations and other global bodies. The independent states in turn align their national policies to the regional priorities set by the regional body. We have to be cognisant of the growing influence of foreign powers interjecting their country's foreign policy agenda's interests into the decision-making process of the Pacific. The Pacific Islands Forum (PIF) – established in 1971 – is the foremost and oldest political forum in the region. The Pacific Islands Development Forum (established in 2012) brings together the public, private and civil society sectors for action promoting sustainable development in the Pacific. The Council of Regional Organisations of the Pacific (CROP) provides educational, scientific and technical support to the Forum Leaders and assists in policy development and implementation in the region. The Pacific Islands Association of Non-Government Organisation (PIANGO) is a regional organisation consisting of NGOs in 22 Pacific Island countries. PIANGO critically looks at Pacific Island Forums Leaders' policies and initiatives, participates in the consultation processes of the region and in 2018 was granted consultative status to the United Nations Economic and Social Council (Pacific Islands Association of Non-government Organisations, 2018). The Secretariat of Pacific Community, commonly known as SPC or Pacific Community, is also active in providing regional efforts in the sciences including health and social development. There are also three ecumenical religious organisations – Pacific Conference of Churches (PCC), Pacific Theological College (PTC) and the South Pacific Association of Theological Schools (SPATS). Each of these organisations plays a significant role in the spiritual and religious life of Pacific societies and communities and are actively involved in societal issues of regional concern.

The Pacific region is perceived to be dependent on foreign aid and the reliance on international development assistance is seen to be a feature of Pacific Island economies into the future (Pryke, 2013). Hau'ofa (1994), however, argues that such perceptions inadequately account for the resourcefulness which comes from Pacific peoples and cultures. Nonetheless, evidence suggests that China has become a major player in providing various forms of assistance and loans to Pacific countries which furthers the strategic goals of China's foreign policy in the Pacific and increases debt to China as well as being a counteraction to Taiwanese influence. The Australian Government announced in November 2018 that it would create a multi-billion dollar fund for infrastructure development in the Pacific "in an apparent attempt to counter China's influence" (BBC, 2018). However, research indicates that debt in the region is a problem but that it is "not debt to China that is of concern" (Pryke, 2013). Social service provision within the Pacific is substantively influenced by international donor-funding and social workers need to critically reflect on the impacts of this context on practice.

Pacific social work is inclusive of local and broader social issues that are prevalent across our communities. Critical challenges facing Pacific nations and communities include: The Pacific has 6 of the 15 countries most vulnerable to climate change in the world; the cost of natural disasters to GDP include Fiji (30%) and Vanuatu (64%); youth unemployment averages 23% in the Pacific compared to the global average of 13%; there are high rates of non-communicable diseases, which is the cause of 84% of deaths in Fiji; traditional forms of social protection are increasingly under threat (Pacific Islands Forum Secretariat, 2018). Human rights in the region focusing on the indigeneity and self-determination for the peoples of Tannah (West) Papua controlled by Indonesia is another issue relevant to social work. The decolonisation of Kanaky (New Caledonia) and Maòhi Nui (French Polynesia) from France has been side-tracked by the governments of the region except for the persistent stance of the Government of Vanuatu. These issues have been taken up by the NGO and faith-based sectors. Redress and compensation for the health and environmental impacts of the effects of nuclear testing by France in Maòhi Nui (French Polynesia) is another issue of concern. Food security concerns across the Pacific has arisen as a result of rising sea levels brought on by climate change, overfishing of community fishing grounds by foreign fishing vessels and concerns around the environmental impact of seabed and deep sea bed mining. Of course, these seem scientific in nature, but have a major flow onto the social, in which Pacific social work should concern itself on and around. It is important to recognise that many of the social issues facing Pacific peoples have roots in the colonisation project. For example, personal and structural racism experienced by Pacific peoples, whether in their homelands or in the diaspora, can be perceived as remnants of the "blackbirding" era where Pacific peoples were taken as slaves to aid European profiteering (Speedy, 2015).

Traditionally, the dominant way of looking at the Pacific has been through an economic lens, where financially they are dependent on foreign aid and goodwill due to their lack of industry and trade. However, it is within this deficit view that continues to undermine the resilience and pioneering spirit that has governed the Islands for centuries. Rather than perceiving Pacific perspectives as being viable and valid, they are relegated as archaic and outmoded to the detriment of then upholding indigenous knowledge as key to Pacific wellbeing. Colonial and westernised ways of knowing, doing, being and becoming are then traded for these strong collectivist values and beliefs, creating ongoing tensions across our Pacific region and the Pacific diaspora striving to also uphold their traditional approaches.

Terms to describe Pacific peoples are varied, reflecting both the geo-political context and the fluidity of Pacific identities (Tupuola, 2004). Table 1.1 highlights words commonly utilised to describe Pacific people, along with a meaning and comments on the context-specific fluidity of its application. The applications show the complexity inherent in labels of identity. It is important for

TABLE 1.1 Terms to describe Pacific people

Term	Meaning	Application
Pacific	People that originate from across the Pacific Region – including Polynesia, Melanesia and Micronesia.	Used to describe Pacific communities from the Pacific region (including Indigenous peoples and descendants of indentured labourers) and peoples of Pacific ethnicities across the diaspora globally.
Pacific Islander	People that originate from across the Pacific Region – including Polynesia, Melanesia and Micronesia.	Used to describe those originating from the Islands. In New Zealand, it is not inclusive of Māori. In Papua New Guinea, "highlanders" and "islanders" are differentiated based on which areas of the country they are from. Therefore, those from the highlands and in-land regions do not identify with this term, but they are considered "Pacific islanders" by mainstream society when in Australia, New Zealand or the USA.
Pasifika	Cultural term used to describe Pacific Islanders and their traditional practices.	Used in New Zealand and Australia to refer to Pacific peoples living there and their cultures. In New Zealand, however, the term excludes Māori given their status as Indigenous, rather than migrant, in that context.
Islander	Abbreviated terminology referring to Pacific Islanders and their cultures	When referring to certain practices or perspectives, foods or approaches.

social workers to demonstrate flexibility and skill to work with multiple layers of identity (Nadan, 2017), according to how one positions themselves in relation to nationality, island, village, culture and language. This is especially so in urban settings and in the diaspora where there are increasing numbers of people with mixed-Pacific ethnicity and the degree of Pacific mobility across the region and globe.

We understand the importance of using terminology that is socially just which can also captivate and richly define the complexities associated with Pacific ancestry and its multifaceted traditions. Therefore, we as editors have consciously chosen to use the phrase *Pacific* to capture our desire to ensure our community is positioned in a helpful way. We believe the notion of *Pacific* is rooted in the collective, positioning people in purpose and place. That is, the *Pacific* represents a shared locality; with the vast array of Islands and countries united through the Pacific Ocean. Despite the many differences that occur across the seas, we share a common love for the way in which Pacific cultures have been shaped and transformed by its inextricable connection to the land and its surrounding waters. Over time, this has yielded a close connection with subsistent lifestyles across this locality, with views that others who also share the same Island are also connected through a similar respect and approach. As Pacific people have moved to other places across the region, including places like Australia, USA and Europe, they may use this shared understanding of who they are in their new homelands, clinging closely with traditional practices to remind them of who they are, where they come from and what they represent. This is manifested through the celebration and use of language, further highlighted through songs, dances, poetry and storytelling.

Therefore, this notion of sharing within a collectivist approach to how we are connected also assists Pacific people to understand their place in the world. Positionality in where we are physically located can also impact on the way in which we perceive social and welfare needs and the way in which we strive to resolve such matters. This can include whether we are Pacific-born or are part of the diaspora elsewhere to those that have migrated to the Pacific and the knowledge created and developed through owning such spaces and places.

Perspectives and practice

Considering Pacific people have a specific space and place, also influenced in a contemporary context by the realities of globalism, it is important now as ever to position these notions of Pacific in the context of practice. Rather than implementing strategies that are only defined by dominant discourses generally determined by the *global north*, Pacific people and the region we occupy should also inform the various approaches undertaken across contemporary social structures. This includes the need to understand the role of Pacific perspectives in the vast field of practices evident across this book. And this is where such intersections occur; each author involved in contributing to their chapter is writing from this space, striving to promote a greater understanding of what Pacific as practice would look like. The ability to bring over 30 contributors to provide a rigorous review of areas that concern our Pacific people is also evident of the need to inform practice through and via a Pacific lens.

This book is also aspiring to create an idea of evolving models of practice that have previously been established by and for Pacific people. That is, the ability to now extend and build upon Pacific models that have been postulated, developed and implemented is also occurring. It is within this context that we see Pacific as not being a static area of practice, but instead a vibrant and ever-changing process that is still underpinned by the richness that represents the Pacific. This includes ensuring that the chapters are providing a broader understanding of social and welfare issues across the micro, meso and macro, enabling a local, regional and international understanding. From this approach, we strive to ensure that a shared understanding of such need through the inclusion of many Pacific states and territories across Oceania and beyond, whilst also profiling the many strengths found within the Pacific are utilised as part of the desire to create a collaboratively and shared response.

We acknowledge that this book in its entirety is also striving to promote an ongoing local, regional and international conversation about the importance of decolonising professional practice, including social work. As a growing trend is happening globally across many disciplines, the main driver is counteracting the harmful effects of privileging certain ideas as being the right fit for all, rather than appreciating the cohesion that comes from including cultural diversity and its differences. This includes the need to understand differences based on ethnicity and indigeneity, but also rightly applies to differences that occur due to gender, class, religion, sexuality and ability. Hence, the need to create a shared space that is inclusive and communal and collective in its shared narrative and practice. Within this context we believe practice can be influenced by the Pacific and their right to inform and be included in the broader scope and field of social work.

It is part of this bigger picture approach to unpack the various contexts in which Pacific can be applied that we have developed a definition of *Pacific Social Work*. First, through understanding Pacific as a form of perspective, we are promoting a greater positioning of Pacific people, their families and communities as a valid space to work from. Second, through understanding Pacific as geopolitical, we acknowledge the inextricable reality of globalism, its economic and social structures and the need to work within a broader regional context beyond the local level. Bringing this all together is the context of Pacific as practice, where the various fields of social work practice evolve cultural models and approaches.

Conclusion

Within this chapter, we strive to further set a tone around the way in which the concept of Pacific is understood through varying contexts; as a perspective, as geo-politics, as practice and as a form of social work. From this platform comes the ongoing encouragement and desire to ensure Pacific is understood beyond the idyllic tourist destination, to a complex and informed space and place where various aspects of social work can operate in a culturally safe and humble manner.

We hope that by understanding the various contexts of Pacific, social work education, practice, policy and research can continue to be meaningfully developed and implemented that is inclusive and just. We also hope that this book will be the start of an ongoing *talanoa* (conversation) about how this may manifest within social work as a profession across the many spaces and places in which Pacific people occupy, with the view that they are consistently part of the conversation around the changes they may experience within their own social and welfare needs, whilst also creating communities that are informed by culturally relevant perspectives and approaches.

References

BBC. (2018, November). Australia ramps up Pacific spending amid China debate. *BBC World News Australia*. Retrieved from www.bbc.com/news/world-australia-46133560

Garrett, J. (1982). *To live among the stars: Christian origins in Oceania. Geneva and Suva.* (World Council of Churches in association with the Institute of Pacific Studies, Ed.). Suva, Fiji: The University of the South Pacific.

Hau'ofa, E. (1994). Our sea of islands. *The Contemporary Pacific, 6*(1), 148–161.

Hau'ofa, E. (1998). The ocean in us. *The Contemporary Pacific, 10*(2), 391–410.

Ka'ili, T. O. (2017). *Marking indigeneity: The Tongan art of sociospatial relations.* Tucson, AZ: The University of Arizona Press.

Lewis, M. (2018). *Cultural disparity and political solidarity in the Melanesian world.* Retrieved from www.geocurrents.info/geopolitics/cultural-disparity-and-political-solidarity-in-the-melanesian-island-world

Mila, K. (2017). Mana Moana: Healing the va, developing spiritually and culturally embedded practices. In L. Béres (Ed.), *Practising spirituality: Reflections on meaning-making in personal and professional contexts* (pp. 61–71). Basingstoke: Macmillan.

Nadan, Y. (2017). Rethinking "cultural competence" in international social work. *International Social Work, 60*(1), 74–83. https://doi.org/doi:10.1177/0020872814539986

Pacific Islands Association of Non-government Organisations. (2018). *PIANGO receives special UN status.* Retrieved from www.piango.org/uncategorized/piango-receives-special-un-status/

Pacific Islands Forum Secretariat. (2018). First quadrennial Pacific sustainable development report: Executive summary. Retrieved from Suva, Fiji: www.forumsec.org/wp-content/uploads/2018/09/1st-Quadrennial-Pacific-Sustainable-Development-Report-2018.pdf

Pryke, J. (2013). *Rising aid dependency in the Pacific.* Retrieved from www.devpolicy.org/rising-aid-dependency-in-the-pacific-20130917/

Speedy, K. (2015). The Sutton case: The first Franco-Australian foray into blackbirding. *Journal of Pacific History, 50*(3), 344–364.

Tupuola, A. M. (2004). Pasifika edgewalkers: Complicating the achieved identity status in youth research. *Journal of Intercultural Studies, 25*(1), 87–100. https://doi.org/doi:10.1080/07256860410001687045

2
CONTEMPORARY PACIFIC VALUES AND BELIEFS

Aliitasi Su'a-Tavila

Key points

- Embracing both traditional and contemporary Pacific values and beliefs can inform effective social work with Pacific people.
- Specific roles and responsibilities within the cultural context will impact the way in which cultural practices are upheld and implemented.
- Notions of living a life in service to others underpins communal perspectives, which can also permeate the role of Pacific social work in and across the community.

Introduction

It is how we grew up in our individual environment that gives us understanding of this world. It is how we understand the world around us that influences our actions. It is our actions and reactions that bring outcomes. It is how we interpret outcomes that enhances new learnings. As Pacific social work practitioners, it is our understanding of Pacific epistemologies that informs our professional practices. What constitutes our philosophical knowing is underpinned in our cultural values and beliefs. This in turn maintains our identity and who we are. Unfortunately, the implications of globalisation and modernisation seem to be the driving forces of many challenges amongst the Pacific people's world. Fortunately, Pacific people's persistence to hold onto their culture enables them to evolve with the modern world despite numerous challenges. One of the challenges noted is the dilution of traditional characteristics within our social structures. One example is the transition from communal society to urban society and from extended family to nuclear family. Notwithstanding the challenges we encounter, one of the coping mechanisms that sustains us in the new environment is our cultural and collective approach.

The dichotomy of traditional and contemporary world views that challenges our thinking does matter when we work with communities experiencing conditions which create vulnerabilities in a social work context. While the concept of "social work" has informally existed across the Pacific through cultural practices and responsibilities, the value of our traditional daily practice at home, in a village and in church communities remains resilient within us. Essentially, these traditional practices influence our holistic understanding of the world and gives us insight about what Pacific social work practice might look like in the contemporary world. Though each Pacific Island nation is unique in its own right, there are some similarities relative to our history and genealogy that affirms the shared nature of our designation and identity. Thus, it modifies social work practice within the Pacific community globally. Our traditional practice and how it informs our contemporary approach to professional practice is crucial (Ravulo, 2016; Sua-Tavila, 2010). Within the context of this work, traditional practice is a cultural-based practice where the service provided is founded on cultural norms that are appropriate when working alongside individuals, families, communities and societies. For instance, working with Samoan families, the concept of *fa'aaloalo* is common to the discussion/dialogue and its application to the practical knowledge is relevant. Similarly, from a Tongan perspective, Mafile'o (2006) highlights the value of *kainga* (family). The concept of *Kainga* is central to Tongan social work practice because it stands as a philosophical template for relationship building and meaning in the interface between social workers and their clients. Utilising the concept of *kainga* provides theoretical insights of social work practice when working with the Tongan community.

The significance of upholding cultural beliefs that determines our thinking around a strategic approach to today's social work practice is relevant to the discussion. This chapter profiles these important concepts and concludes with discussions about the value of embracing both traditional and contemporary thinking when practicing social work within the Pacific community. Particular attention is given to structural thinking and how it enhances our service as Pacific social workers.

Pacific epistemology: A Samoan perspective

The continuous practice around daily lifestyle as well as traditional protocols are pertinent to most Pacific customs and is informed by various Pacific epistemologies. Subsequently, it becomes a norm to generations after generations who grew up in their village and family environment without realisation. The complexity of Pacific epistemologies within the Pacific is acknowledged, however, an example from Samoa is discussed to provide another perspective and to demonstrate its relevance to social work practice. This epistemology is called "*aga-i-fanua*", (rule of the land). Different traditional protocols and rules in the Samoan families and villages are known as *aga-i-fanua*, meaning there are particular customs relevant to an individual family or village according to its history and genealogy

(Efi, 2007). The epistemological perception within *aga-i-fanua* offers a basic explanation of some traditional methods to justify its imperative in relation to Pacific social work practice. Tui Atua Tupua Tamasese Taisi Efi (2007) explains the *aga-i-fanua* concept as a rule or law which specifically applies to a family or a village and its origins in history and genealogy. Some villages have special roles afforded to particular families, names or positions specific to their village history. This specificity is privileged in the operations and imperatives of *aga-i-fanua* and recorded in village *fa'alupega* (or chiefly honorifics) (p. 7).

Philosophically, the concept of *aga-i-fanua* takes us to another level of cultural understanding as it underpins our way of knowing. *Aga-i-fanua* recognises the uniqueness of each village and family and it is through observations and practices that one would gain knowledge and learn the in-depth meaning of *aga-i-fanua*. The specifics of *aga-i-fanua* are reference points for discussion amongst families and village people when serious matters occur either at home, in a village or in the community at large. It has explicit connections to the building of kinship amongst *aiga* (family) and *nuu* (village); thus, its epistemological stance symbolises meaningful Samoan values, beliefs and practices. The exclusive elements of *aga-i-fanua* are the very essence of social work practice when working with Samoans and also with relevance to other Pacific groups. These are *fa'aaloalo* (respect) and *va fealoaloa'i* (respectful relationship). These values are very comprehensive when practising *fa'a-Samoa* in various contexts. Drawing on these values within a social work context informs our world view on what, when and how we integrate the *aga-i-fanua* specifics to nurture those who are considered vulnerable to the global changes and eventually become our social work clients.

The ritual of exercising *aga-i-fanua* concepts is immense when critical situations happen in Samoan families. Its application involves consultations held by family leaders to ensure the process brings positive outcomes. From experience and observations, understanding *aga-i-fanua* within a family and village context may potentially lead to overcoming challenges facing young generations because of western influence that may contradict their own traditional characteristics. The following case study illustrates how the values of *aga-i-fanua* has informed a decision to address a serious situation that disturbed peace in the village context.

CASE STUDY 2.1

In one particular nuu (village), the prohibition of planting, selling or consumption of cannabis and any other outlawed drugs is common knowledge. Everyone is aware of this rule and the village protocol and anyone who breaches it faces severe punishment. Two residents brought this contraband into the nuu environment hoping that the village council would be none the wiser. It was only when a man uncharacteristically threatened to kill his wife that his family discovered that he had acted under the influence

> of a hallucinatory substance. The village council was informed immediately and an emergency meeting was convened within the hour to deal with this breach. The village council ruling resulted in the permanent banishment from the village of both the seller and the consumer. These offenders were given 10 hours to vacate the village or their homes inhabited not only by themselves but by the members of their respective family would be set alight.

Traditionally, the village jurisdiction system was already in place many years ago and it was followed accordingly. The situation was dealt with by the council of chiefs immediately via their *fono* (meeting) without anyone's interference. The village *fono* are conducted without minute taking and points of discussion are communicated orally. It has its own unique structure of addressing issues because the law of the land is understood by all. Thus, the purpose of the urgent *fono* was to determine the severity of the offence and the appropriate penalty to counteract the behaviour. The prohibition of drugs in the village environment is a rule set by leaders to prevent harm. *Aga-i-fanua* ideology prevents external influence to be introduced in the village. Regardless of any offence committed by village people, it is the village's *aga-i-fanua* to impose punishment for those who disrupt justice, peace and harmony; in particular, situations where violence occurs amongst families as it is considered a disrespectful and uncivilised action. The family's decision to inform the council of chiefs about the problem suggests their respect of the village *aga-i-fanua* as it is part of the village protocol to report any mischievous activity happening inside the village.

History expresses that the value of *aga-i-fanua* defines our designation, and when it is violated, there is a particular process to employ. However, each village adopts its own process based on their *aga-i-fanua*. Unlike the western approach of dealing with criminal cases, where the process could be prolonged and involve various levels of discussion, the traditional approach to address the violation of *aga-i-fanua* is somewhat unique. It is based on traditional protocols set by the ancestors and governed by the leaders. The values of *fa'aloalo* and *va fealoaloa'i* are critical to the process because it has implications on both the village and the family involved. From the family's viewpoint, it has an impact on the whole family and they (family) have a responsibility to demonstrate the value of *va fealoaloa'i* by providing food to feed the village to maintain their dignity and keep the family safe. From the village's viewpoint, it is their responsibility to practice disciplinary actions and to intervene to address inappropriate behaviour at all times. Thus, the consequence was more a response to the values of *aga-i-fanua* being diminished rather than the actual offence.

Drawing from the traditional practice of addressing inappropriate behaviour, the significance of *aga-i-fanua* is embraced by two values of *fa'aaloalo* and *va fealoaloa'i*. Relative to contemporary social work practice, *aga-i-fanua* values inform alternative interventions to engage with Pacific communities and in particular the Samoan community. It provides another lens for the social work practitioners to *talanoa* with the family/individual and bring meaningful insights into the conversation. While the village has fulfilled its protocols to impose penalties on offenders, there is also a process in place to restore a relationship with the offenders. The common one is a reciprocity process where a family and a village council *talanoa* to address and agree on resolutions appropriate to various cases.

The epistemological approach of *aga-i-fanua* defines who we are in our traditional world. It informs our contemporary knowing when dealing with Pacific families as it symbolises family, village and a societal sense of belonging and identity. The philosophical approach of *aga-i-fanua* enhances our social work practical thinking when we encounter clients at a micro, meso and macro level of the society. Understanding *aga-i-fanua* principles and its application to our social work practice illustrate the notion of cultural awareness and appropriateness when we engage with the Samoan community and other Pacific groups across the board. For Pacific social workers, it is our pride to carry our own *aga-i-fanua* which in turn illustrates our status and relationship with others. Fundamental to the practice of *aga-i-fanua* is the provision of service within various contexts to ensure cultural values and beliefs are strengthened. The provision of this service is called *tautua*.

The epistemological value of *tautua* (service) as a social work imperative

Tautua is a significant element of *fa'a-Samoa*. It is a unique service that underpins one's responsibility to serve accordingly at home, a village and church. The most obvious point of reference to the *tautua* concept in the *fa'a-Samoa* is between a *taule'ale'a* (untitled man) and his *matai* (chief) and the entire family. The *taule'ale'a* provides an efficient service for his family in one of the most demanding jobs in *fa'a-Samoa* because *tautua* is considered tough, challenging and sometimes dangerous. The word *tautua* is a combination of two syllables that reveal its depth of meaning. These are *tau* and *tua*. *Tau* literally means "fight", however, within the context of providing a service, *tau* means "work" or "serve". *Tua* literally means "back" or "behind", hence the word *tautua* means "work from the back" or "serve from behind". Through *tautua*, the *taule'ale'a* has a firm belief that the provision of service will earn blessings from the receivers or consumers of the service. These blessings act as ongoing fortune for the family in the future. One example is that the recognition of one's ability to provide service brings great rewards as in the Samoan saying *'O le ala i le pule o le tautua*. This brief Samoan saying stipulates the crucial element of *tautua* (service) where one has to endure painful experiences to serve their family with commitment, trust and humility for a certain length of time in order to become a *matai* (title male) which holds status in the family environment. The extent and the success of *tautua* demonstrates one's ability to lead the family in the future and to represent the family in the village council forums. It legitimises the practice of work from behind the scene for the benefit of the family. The potential consequences of providing poor *tautua* could shift the family status because of its economic impact.

The epistemological value of *tautua* in *fa'a-Samoa* is the provision of quality services that comes with a positive outcome. It is a service that is learned through observations, experience and practice. A quality service principle resonates social work practice in terms of providing good service to social work clients with the intention of positive outcomes. Furthermore, when providing *tautua* it is an alternative approach to make changes for their own (client) benefit. The *taule'ale'a's* commitment to provide the best service to his *aiga* to sustain and maintain their welfare and wellbeing corresponded to the approach relevant to social work practice with reference to the provision of good service to our client. It is a commitment that we learn through practice, observations, experience and service. Ebacher (2013) argues that service learning is based on the assumption that knowledge is obtained in the interactive process of actions and reflections and it benefits the served community. However, the practising of the service can be varied according to the context; hence the implications can be different. The effectiveness of interactions between the social worker and their clients depends on the extent of knowledge, skill and experience gained. As an outcome, the magnitude of service provided is different. According to Barreneche and Ramos-Flores (2013), service learning is a pedagogy and an effective vehicle for teaching students about citizenship and civic engagement. Likewise, another epistemological value of *tautua* is a service that is practiced from the heart and it is embraced with the cultural values of *fa'aaloalo* and *va fealoaloa'i*. These are the imperatives of social work practice embedded in the *fa'a-Samoa* without realisation. The *tautua* concept is manifested in the traditional daily practice and in turn informs our contemporary thinking as social work practitioners. Relationship building and community connection through services provided by social work practitioners increases a sense of responsibility for our clients.

Overall, *tautua* through *taule'ale'a* as a social work imperative is a reciprocal process that enriches the trust between the service provider and the recipient. It is a form of power and identity that is embraced with love, respect and trust. It is a service that is provided with the belief of obtaining blessings from the recipient of the service and the expectation that generations to come will harvest the blessings. It is through observing, learning, experience and reflection that service can be recognised and the outcome of the service recognition is the bestowment of the *matai* title (either chief or an orator) which is an honour to attain. From experience, to achieve set goals that promote changes in a client's situation when working in a social work context is considered a blessing. It is a service well provided that benefits clients.

E sui faiga ae tumau fa'avae (the form changes but the founding principles of *fa'a-Samoa* remains)

E sui faiga ae tumau fa'avae is a Samoan idiom that depicts the philosophical view that the transformation of modern thinking to our cultural norms when traditional practices are implemented does not change the principles that underpin the essence of practice. Fundamentally, the relevance of the Samoan idiom to a social work context informs our approach when we engage with our own people. Understanding that Pacific diasporic communities in New Zealand are rapidly increasing helps to also understand the changing dynamics around the social issues they encounter. Thus, blending new knowledge and thinking to our traditional knowing substantiates our practice in the social work realm. Explicably, ideas and ideologies learned from exposure to different cultures enhances new changes. Eventually these new changes are incorporated into the individual's traditional norms without attention and could be viewed as a cultural divide. MacPherson and MacPherson (2009) refer to cultural divide as a split between what is indigenous and what is not. Acknowledging the aspect of cultural divide allows room to enhance contemporary knowledge. When addressing issues pertaining to Samoan people in New Zealand, drawing on the values of *fa'aaloalo* and *va fealoaloa'i* has a more substantive impact rather than focusing on contemporary approaches alone. The *fa'a-Samoa* principle and its cultural values to be integrated into the discussion could influence the outcome one way or the other. While the growing diversity of the Pacific population globally brought various perspectives, it is how we understand the practical application of our service to whom we engage with. Equally important is how we as social work practitioners see the founding principles fit within our practice. From a Pacific perspective, providing service is fundamental to our daily activities without realising it correlates to social work practice. Understanding the appropriateness of Pacific epistemologies values allows us to adapt our practice in various contexts. Reflecting on the values of *fa'a-Samoa* within the context of social work in the contemporary world are the imperatives relevant to social work practice.

The cultural practice within the context of village and family is basically the same in terms of it being governed by the *pule-fa'amatai* (chiefly authority). From the village approach, it is governed by the council of chiefs and from an individual family approach it is governed by the family chief.

Traditional worldviews and contemporary social work practices hold hands: A Samoan perspective

Pacific people's origin is well-argued and explained in the literature. Although the work of early Pacific scholars started to indigenise Pacific knowledge, this was not enough to give recognition to indigenous thoughts from an academic point of view (Huffer & Qalo, 2004). Furthermore, Huffer and Qalo argue that the lack of a coherent voice to promote Pacific thought or philosophy means our world view is also diminished. Historically, the common perception of Pacific people's designation are people from the ocean. They are navigators, sea farers and storytellers. Despite this generalisation, Pacific people's cultural values and beliefs are complex, unique and somehow similar. One of the similarities observed is their communal lifestyle. The value of communal lifestyles cannot be underestimated as it embeds cultural protocols and norms.

For example, the dynamics of *fa'a-Samoa* remains static throughout historical interventions from colonialists and early foreigners in the 19th century despite their many efforts to change it. One must understand that the strength of *fa'a-Samoa* lies within its communal approach led by the *pule fa'amatai* (chiefly authority). The chiefly authority has enormous influence over the village community as well as individual families. It is the governing system that is exercised by the council of chiefs who controls a village's daily affairs that influence the family environment. Within the village context, communal lifestyle means a collective approach to do various tasks that benefits everyone under the council of chiefs' leadership. A village is a community of different *aiga* (family) within a certain locality. A council of chiefs is a combination of individual family chiefs who are representatives of their families and can be ranked from paramount chiefs, chiefs and orators. It holds the highest rank in the village structure and they are the decision and policy makers of the village. Interestingly, historians and anthropologists view Samoa's chiefly system as a unique cultural heritage of Samoa (Meleisea, 1987). Its dominant nature has successfully maintained its indigenous culture for many centuries. Their leadership is complex as it is intrinsically woven into the fabric of Samoan culture and history. The practising of their authority is underpinned by the notion of love, respect and caring. When serious problems occur, they are the immediate mediators, counsellors and advisors, to name a few, because they are considered a safety net; hence their authority is seldom challenged by anyone. For that reason, they receive an ultimate respect from everyone in the village. They regularly monitor the village community through their monthly meetings to ensure that everyone is constantly alert to the village protocols to prevent unnecessary problems that may disturb the village community. Consequences are imposed to those who dispute or disobey the village protocols. One example of some village protocols is that women are forbidden to wear long pants as it is considered culturally inappropriate. Village people view it as a western style and it does not fit within their traditional fashion. These are some of the cultural understandings that provide meaning and insight into our professional daily practice. It also endorses the significance of village traditions that have been preserved by the forefathers and the practices that have continued through many generations.

The inheritance of *fa'a-Samoa* cultural values and beliefs as well as a communal approach substantiate our practical thinking around social work context. The notion of blending traditional norms into a contemporary approach does strengthen the process of working with Samoan clients in a multi-cultural environment. For example, Mulitalo-Lauta (2000) developed a model called Lalaga Model. Lalaga means weave or plait. According to Mulitalo-Lauta (2000), the philosophical basis of this integrated model derives from *fa'a-Samoa* on the one hand, and from the adopted contemporary culture (Western) on the other. It emphasises the principle of partnership and the need for the social worker to practice in a bicultural framework, that is the *fa'a-Samoa* and the contemporary adopted culture of Aotearoa/New Zealand. In the contemporary setting of Aotearoa/New Zealand, the use of *pandanas* leaves symbolises the weaving together of two cultural elements from both Samoa and Aotearoa/New Zealand within the social work context.

Communal approach in the family context is similar to the village context except it is considered a linear version. The Samoan family context is a combination of a *matai* (family chief) and his *aiga* who are both functioned together and one cannot be fully appreciated and comprehended without the other. Traditionally, the *matai*, who is always a male, is the head of the family. From experience, he is the sole decision-maker and receives full support from his *aiga*. The *aiga* is the core unit of Samoan social life and it is considered an initial platform to learn the essence of *fa'a-Samoa* and how it operates. Grattan (1985) notes that the *aiga* is the pillar of the Samoan political organisation. The *matai* is the head of the *aiga* who is responsible for the welfare and wellbeing of his *aiga* socially, culturally and spiritually. Kamu (2003) provided a definition of the Samoan *aiga*:

> *Aiga* is not limited to the primary family of parents and children or a married couple with no children. It includes a wider family group of blood and marriage relations, in-laws and their families, and even those who may not be related as such. It includes persons who have little, if any blood connection but who have been adopted into it, not by any process of law but merely by the kindly local custom which ensures that no person shall be homeless. It includes all those who have acknowledged the leadership of the family *matai*. Members of the aiga do not live in one house or necessarily live in the same village.
>
> (Kamu, 2003, p. 39)

The relationship between the *matai* and his *aiga* is rather strong as it is supported by all family members. Communal approach within the family context means everyone is aware that the *matai* holds the authority to govern the family including the power to distribute family resources and dedicate roles and responsibilities to respective family members. Each family member understands his/her own roles and responsibilities as these are informed by their cultural values and beliefs.

The context of *fa'a-Samoa* is multi-layered and it provides an in-depth knowledge of its relevance to social work practice. It is the social and cultural structure in the *fa'a-Samoa* that informs our epistemological approach to our professional practice. Communal lifestyle to many Samoan people is defined by its social and cultural expectations. This gives reference to their identity and belonging which is underpinned by cultural obligations. Theoretically, the formulation of one's identity is largely influenced by culture and the recognition of a client's history and background enhances thorough assessments and interventions within the social work context.

Conclusion

Working alongside the Pacific community needs an effective social work approach that complements their unique world view. Understanding Pacific epistemologies provide a framework for social workers to recognise the diversity of Pacific people's social environment. Communal approach, *aga-i-fanua* and service learning provides flexibility and creativity with developing an intervention plan when engaged with the Pacific and non-Pacific community and it can add unique strengths to our social work practice approaches, policy and research. From a Samoan perspective, the conceptualising of Pacific epistemologies provides some tools for social work practitioners to enrich their practice. The knowledge shared in this chapter comes from an indigenous Samoan woman who lives and admires her culture and wishes to promote the importance of *fa'a-Samoa* to the generations to come and others. Understanding the correlation between the traditional norm and contemporary context justifies our practice in a diverse environment. In other words, the philosophical underpinnings of our own epistemologies informs our practices in the professional context. It is how we understand the world around us that influences our actions.

REFLECTIVE QUESTIONS

1. What are the challenges of a Samoan epistemological approach to social work practice?
2. Reflecting on a scenario in a village context, what could be done differently to address the issue?

TABLE 2.1 Glossary of Samoan terms used within chapter

Aga-i-fanua	Rule of the land. The term applies to customary specifics applied to a village or a family according to its genealogy and history
Aiga	Family – immediate or extended families and kin group
Fa'aaloalo	Respect – one of the core elements of Samoan culture
Fa'alupega	Honorific – a specific address given to a person according to his/her status at home, village or church
Fa'a-Samoa	Samoan culture, Samoan way
Fono	Meeting
Kainga	Extended family (Tongan)
Matai	Titled head of a Samoan family
Nu'u	Village
Pule fa'a-matai	Chiefly authority who governs the village
Talanoa	Dialogue between two or more people; discussion
Tau	Fight or serve
Taule'ale'a	An untitled male who is a member of the village sector called aumaga (group of untitled men)
Tautua	Service provided to the family by the taule'ale'a
Tua	Back, from behind
Va fealoaloa'i	Respectful relationship between people

References

Barreneche, G. & Ramos-Flores, H. (2013). Integrated or isolated experiences? Considering the role of service-learning in the Spanish language curriculum. *Hispania, 96*(2), 215–228. Retrieved from www.jstor.org/stable/23608322

Ebacher, C. (2013). Taking Spanish into the community: A novice's guide to service-learning. *Hispania, 96*(2), 397–408. Doi:10.1353/hpn.2013.0064

Efi, T. A. T. T. T. (2007). *Samoan jurisprudence and the Samoan Lands and Titles Court: The perspective of a litigant.* Retrieved from www.headofstate.ws/speeches/samoan%20Jurisprudence%20October%2007.pdf

Grattan, F. J. (1985). *Introduction to Samoan customs* (2nd ed.). Auckland, New Zealand: R McMillan.

Huffer, E. & Qalo, R. 2004. Have we been thinking upside-down? The contemporary emergence of Pacific theoretical thought. *The Contemporary Pacific, 16*(1), 87–116.

Kamu, L. (2003). *The Samoan culture and the Christian gospel.* Samoa: Manfleet Printing.

MacPherson, C. & MacPherson, L. (2009). *The warm winds of change. Globalisation in contemporary Samoa.* Auckland, New Zealand: Auckland University Press.

Mafile'o, T. (2006). Matakäinga (behaving like family): The social worker-client relationship in Pasifika social work. *Social Work Review,* (6), 31–36.

Meleisea, M. (1987). *The making of modern Samoa: Traditional authority and colonial administration in the modern history of Western Samoa.* Fiji: Pacific Studies, University of South Pacific.

Mulitalo-Lauta, P. T. (2000). *Fa'asamoa and social work within the New Zealand context.* Palmerston North, New Zealand: Dunmore Press.

Ravulo, J. (2016). Pacific epistemologies in professional social work practice, policy and research. *Asia Pacific Journal of Social Work and Development, 26*(4), 191–202. Doi:10.1080/02185385.2016.1234970

Su'a-Tavila, A. (2010). *Addressing cultural barriers to enhance the promotion of healthy eating within the Samoan community* (PhD thesis, Victoria University of Wellington, 2010).

3

PACIFIC-INDIGENOUS SOCIAL WORK THEORIES AND MODELS

Tracie Mafile'o, Jean Mitaera and Karlo Mila

Key points

- Pacific-Indigenous social work theories and models, including formal practice theory and other knowledges, provide an alternative to approaches which dominate contemporary practice in the Pacific region and elsewhere.
- Pacific-Indigenous social work theories and models can be mapped according to function (explanation or behaviour change) and level of abstraction (high, mid, low).
- *Turanga Māori* is a Cook Islands conceptual framework transforming family violence and restoring wellbeing comprising: *Akono'anga Māori*, Cook Islands culture; *No teia tuatau*, of this time; and *Tā'anga'anga'ia*, put to practice.
- *Mana Moana* is an approach to healing drawing on generative words, images, metaphors proverbs, narratives from "Oceania's library".

Introduction

> Parallel to us as we drove swam three dolphins. They rose in unison out the water three times before disappearing ... After a long family meeting, three major resolutions were made ... We all knew that it would be so because of the sign we had received earlier.
>
> *(Newport, 2001, p. 8)*

Pacific social work draws on Pacific-Indigenous knowledge, ways of knowing, skills and ways of being. Beyond being social work with Pacific peoples as "clients" or social work practice taking place in a South Pacific locale, Pacific social work is that which draws from knowledge, skills and values deeply rooted in ethnic specific Pacific-Indigenous worldviews.

This chapter introduces Pacific theories and models of social work as a collective body of work inclusive of written, formal Pacific practice theory recognisable to the Western scientific tradition, alongside knowledge and ethics sourced within Pacific oral traditions, connections with the natural environment, the spiritual dimension, lived experiences and practice wisdom. In overviewing Pacific social work practice theories and models, the chapter brings to light the complexities and possibilities presented in the interface of diverse knowledges (Durie, 2004; Weaver, 2015) for Pacific social work practice. The chapter commences with the history of the development of Pacific-Indigenous theories and models for social work. The conceptualisation of Pacific-Indigenous theories and models in relation to other social work knowledge is explored next. Two Pacific practice approaches are then presented: Turanga Maori (Cook Islands) and Mana Moana (pan-Pacific).

The history of Pacific theories and models of social work and why they are important

Social work theories and models are socially constructed (Payne, 2014). Historical, cultural, political and social contexts shape theory. In this sense, all social work theory is an expression of "culture". Within the Pacific diaspora, as populations have diversified, the emergence of Pacific theories and models of social work presents a disruption to the dominant discourses of the profession. Social work has been complicit in colonialism (Johnson & Yellow Bird, 2012) and professional imperialism has characterised the export of social work into "developing" contexts (Midgley, 1981). The combination of social work's Euro-Western roots, contemporary neo-liberalism and right-wing populism (Ife, 2018) results in the dominance of individual casework approaches over neighbourhood collective action and formulaic technocratic responses over holistic integration of the social, emotive, political and spiritual in social work practice. Theories and models socially constructed from Pacific-Indigenous perspectives offer an alternative in which social work is premised on concepts such as (radical) love, relationships and humility (Mafile'o, 2019, in press).

Pacific theories and models of social work are not at all new, although they are "new" to the literature in recent decades. Decoloniality (Walter, 2013) invites the perspective that "social work" is embedded within Oceania social and cultural systems which predate the establishment of the profession within Western contexts. Pacific kinship systems and communal cultures incorporate processes, ethics, knowledge and skills which facilitate the various social work discourses (Mafile'o, 2005) of healing, social order and social change (Payne, 2014). Yet, in the Pacific region there remains a predominance of Western theoretical models and assessment tools in social work (Shek, Golightley & Holloway, 2017). Furthermore, most of the Pacific social work literature has emanated from the Pacific diaspora (such as Pacific writers in New Zealand or the USA), reflecting where the development of and resourcing for the profession is located.

There are calls for stronger alliances between social work development in the diaspora and social development initiatives within Pacific Island homelands (Mafile'o & Vakalahi, 2018). The challenge lies in negotiating ethnic-specific Pacific knowledge, wisdom and ways within a globalised profession in diverse Pacific settings and where Pacific Island nation social service agencies are largely funded by international donors.

In recent decades, Pacific-Indigenous social work approaches have been added to the literature and some formal social work services are explicitly informed by Pacific-Indigenous approaches (for example: Autagavaia, 2001; Child Youth and Family, 2015; Crichton-Hill, 2018; Faleolo, 2009; Mafile'o, 2004; Meo-Sewabu, 2015; Mila-Schaaf, 2006; Mila, 2017; Mulitalo-Lauta, 2000; Pulotu-Endemann, 2001; Ravulo, 2016, 2019; Vakalahi & Godinet, 2014). Across the entire Pacific sector, we are witnessing a renaissance and vitalisation of an indigenous ethic of care sourced to the Pacific region. There have been a plethora of models, metaphors and cultural modes of delivery which are all attempting to do the same thing. They may be pan-Pacific or ethnic-specific, but they are trying to articulate our Pacific point of difference. They are trying to bring the best of us into contemporary Western-dominated working worlds. Each metaphor, each model is an attempt to open a portal into another worldview – an ancestral world – where we healed people very differently. This was – it is undeniable from the literature – holistic, intergenerational, spiritual, ecological, environmental and interpersonal. Pacific-Indigenous social work theories and models, through the use of metaphors and Pacific languages, elevate Pacific cultural ways of practising. As a collective body of work, Pacific-Indigenous approaches centre with a context of relationships. Many of the practices – whether it is the use of language of humility, the use of silence or the home visit opted over a telephone call – represent a relational mindfulness; a priming of the relational space in order to speak truthfully into it.

Mapping of Pacific-Indigenous social work theories and models is a useful exercise for understanding what they offer for practice and how they each sit in relation to each other and in relation to non-Pacific theories and models. Figure 3.1 uses the dimensions developed by Coady (2016) as a framework for such mapping of direct practice theory. The framework includes two continuums. The first continuum is whether a theory is focused on describing or explaining human behaviour or is focused on facilitating change in behaviour. The second is whether the theory's level of abstraction is high, middle or low. Ecological Systems Theory, for example, which has been described as a meta-theory for social work (Nash, O'Donoghue & Munford, 2005), is explanatory and high level; we would similarly place frameworks such as *Fonofale* (Pulotu-Endemann, 2001) and *Te Whare Tapa Wha* (Durie, 1985, 2011) as explanatory and high level type theory. Models such as *Ho'oponopono*, an Indigenous Hawaiian family conflict resolution model, is more prescriptive for practice, similar to the way the Task Centred Model (Payne, 2014) within social work contains prescribed steps. Pacific-Indigenous perspectives, theories and models resonate with the notion

High-level theories and perspectives	Mid-level theories, models, and therapies	Low-level models and therapies for specific problems and populations	Client-specific practice processes
Fonofale (Pulotu-Endemann, 2001); Te Whare Tapa Wha (Durie, 1994); Pola (Mafile'o, 2008); Tanoa (Meo-Sewabu, 2016)	Lalaga (Mulitalo, 2001); Tanoa Ni Veiqaravi (Ravulo, 2019); Mana Moana (Mila, 2017)	Turanga Maori (James et al., 2012); Vuvale Doke Sautu (Lealea et al., 2012); Koe Fakatupuolamaoui he tau magataoa Niue (Tavelia et al., 2012); Fofola e fala kae talanoa e kainga (Tuinukuafe, 2012); Talanoa ile i'a (Faleolo, 2003); E Kaveinga (Crummer et al., 1998)	Reflective, intuitive-inductive theory building or development for change strategies for unique clients; informed by all levels and types of theory

Emphasis on explanatory function ↕ Emphasis on facilitation of change function

higher ⟷ Level of abstraction ⟷ lower

FIGURE 3.1 Mapping of Pacific social work theories and models.

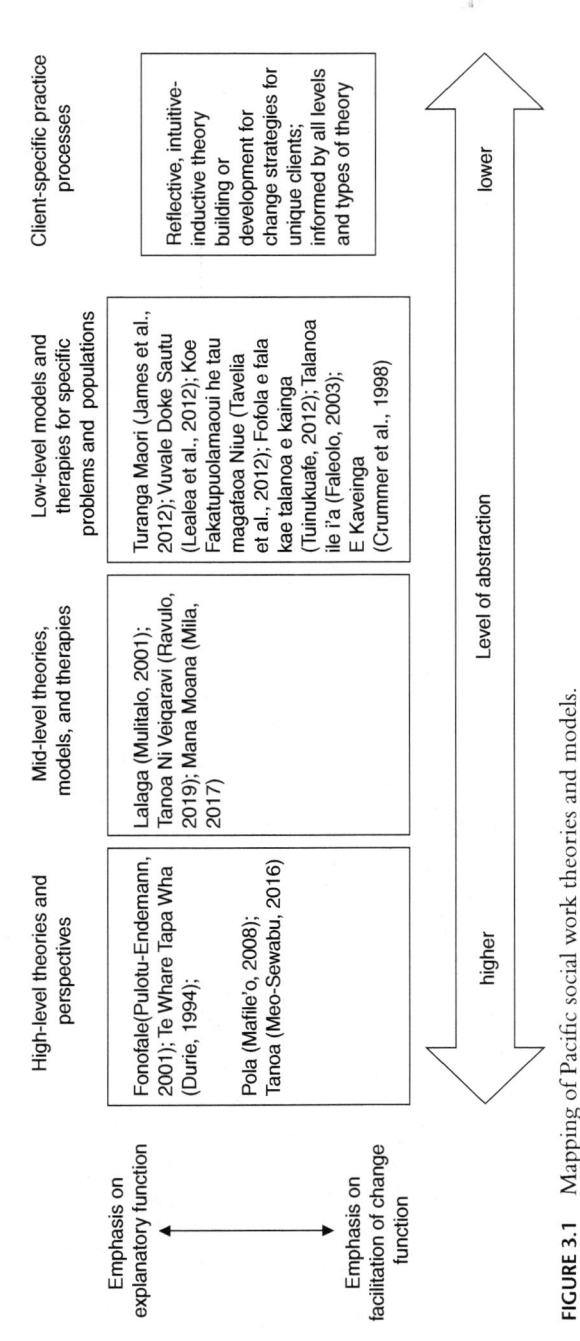

Source: An adaptation of Coady's (2016) function and level of abstraction of theories informing direct social work practice diagram.

of social work as both "science" and "art", and with Coady's (2016) inclusion of reflection, intuition and induction as client-specific practice processes which work alongside high-, mid- and low-level theories and models.

The mapping of selected Pacific social work theory provided in Figure 3.1 demonstrates the tendency of existing formal Pacific theories and models to be explanatory and at a high level of abstraction. This highlights a challenge for Pacific social work practice. While the use of metaphors is empowering, it is also somewhat exclusive. Those who are familiar with the cultural context of the metaphor "know" what the concepts and ideas mean and are more able to intuitively make the application to social work practice. The challenge is to speak to the narrative of the metaphor and to unpack how the concepts, principles and values apply in practice.

Two Pacific-Indigenous direct practice theories and models (*Turanga Māori* and *Mana Moana*), currently utilised in social services with Pacific peoples, are explored next.

Turanga Māori: A Cook Islands conceptual framework transforming family violence – restoring wellbeing

Turanga Māori: A Cook Islands conceptual framework transforming family violence – restoring wellbeing (Ministry of Social Development, 2012) is a Cook Islands response to the increasing number of Cook Islanders affected by family violence. It recognises that Western models have not stemmed the tide of violence and abuse. It is premised on the belief that culture – beliefs, values and knowledges of a people – must inform family violence prevention and intervention strategies. Cook Islands culture, *ākono'anga Māori*, is neither static nor universal; there is no one Cook Islands cultural perspective or practice.

Turanga Māori asserts that all Māori have the right to expect *no'o'anga meitaki* and *ora'anga meitaki*, to live in good circumstances and enjoy a good life. The individual and/or collective has the potential to achieve *ora'anga mou* – live life to the fullest. It assumes a balance of all aspects of life. A good and fulfilled life is acknowledged with the blessing "may you live on", *kia ora ana*. Family violence, abuse, homelessness, trauma, neglect, unwellness and so forth are interruptions to one's wellbeing and disconnect individuals and families from their continuum of wellbeing (see Figure 3.2).

Ora'anga meitaki/ Noo'anga meitaki → To live in good circumstances and enjoy a good life → Ora'anga mou → Live life to the fullest → Kia ora ana → The blessing of a long and fulfilled life

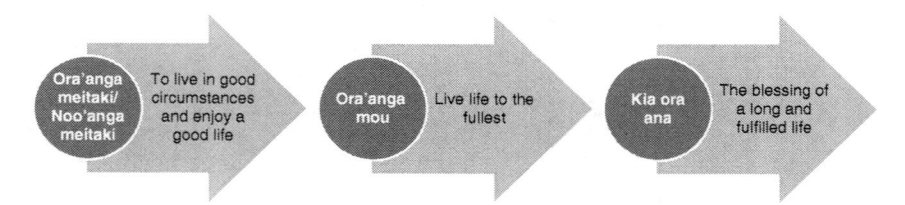

FIGURE 3.2 The continuum of wellbeing.

The three elements of the framework are: (1) *Akono'anga Māori*, Cook Islands culture; (2) *No teia tuatau*, of this time; and (3) *Tā'anga'anga'ia*, put to practice.

1. Akono'anga Māori, Cook Islands culture

Papa'anga, genealogy, is a person's first point of identity, place and responsibilities to self and the collective. This includes *ngutuare tangata* (in relation to household membership), *kopu tangata* (family) and *tapere/vaka* (community).

Turanga refers to position, place and status. All people are born with *turanga* irrespective of gender, order of birth or age. An individual or collective will accumulate *turanga* over time and sometimes relinquish *turanga*. The *turanga* of a first born male is no more important than the *turanga* of a first born daughter – each is born with a distinctive *turanga* and *turanga* in relationship to each other. From a practice perspective, the role of the social worker is to uphold their own professional *turanga* and in their engagement with their Cook Islands client(s) *'akamatūtū i tona turanga* – support the strengthening of his/her position/place/standing, for example, as a father, sister, grandchild or partner. *Turanga* is a good place to start the professional relationship; it is often the place of vulnerability and where a client is most dependent on others.

Piri'anga, relationships and connections, is another aspect of *Akono'anga Māori*. One's *papa'anga* informs on a range of *piri'anga* across generations and between lines of kin. *Piri'anga* affirms *turanga*, *turanga* shapes *piri'anga*. In social work practice, the social worker and the organisation they work for must have robust professional relationships/networks to support their practice – for example, referral agencies, contacts with foodbanks and other support services. When a Cook Islands client is disconnected from their continuum of wellbeing, they are often also disconnected from supportive relationships. The role of the social worker is to support the building of new relationships or the re-building of disconnected relationships. Sometimes it is to assist the client review relationships or make small connections first. *Akamārāmā i tona au piri'anga*, make known his/her relationships/connections. When relationships are established and understood the client is often experiencing their own self-realisation; who they are, who others are and their place within this relationship.

Akaue'anga refers to duties of care and duties to others. Parents have a duty of care for their young children, work colleagues have a duty of care for each other, the taxi driver has a duty of care for his/her passenger and other motorists and good neighbours have a duty of care for each other. The disconnection from one's continuum of wellbeing is often mirrored by the disconnection from duties of care. The strengthening of *turanga* and the re-connecting of relationships brings with it duties of care that need to be exercised. From a cultural perspective, it is this duty of care for others and their duty of care for you that maintains balance and harmony. Practically, the duty may be to maintain contact with a family member, this may not require a home visit, but can be satisfied with a text message. Scale is sometimes worthy of exploration, it is not meant to be a penalty but a developing acknowledgement of co-existence and distinct and shared responsibilities. Distinct, because your duty will be influenced by your *turanga*.

Finally, *ngakau aro'a* is willingness and conviction of the heart, generosity to self and others. It is the emotional and spiritual expression of being Māori. When *turanga, piri'anga* and *akaue'anga* are no longer monitored positions of engagement but free and open expressions of one's "self" we have reached *ngakau aro'a* and transformed from dependence to self-realisation to interdependence. This is the consciousness that "I am part of a whole".

2. No teia tuatau, *of this time*

No teia tuatau, of this time, emphasises the importance of being relevant and realistic given the social, economic, cultural and environmental contexts that people live in today. This aspect is about being mindful that culture/s continue to grow and be shaped by the world within which it exists. People bring their own lived experience and lens to their various situations. When engaging with Cook Islands families, it is important to: (i) *komakoma marie*, let our conversation be unhurried, be in the now; and (ii) *kia maru to korua komakoma'anga*, let your conversations be calm and measured.

3. Tā'anga'anga'ia, *put to practice*

Transformation occurs when *akono'anga Māori*, being relevant to the time and environment, are put into practice. On their own they are simply cultural concepts, isolated in space and without purpose.

Turanga Māori is one conceptual framework. Irrespective of the model or framework a practitioner chooses, the model or framework is but a tool to inform and guide practice. Turanga Māori's purpose is to be relevant and effective for Cook Islands Maori client(s) and practitioners. That practice should be informed by the culture of the people we serve.

Mana Moana

Mana Moana developed out of a search for what is healing in Pacific mental health (Mila, 2017). It has been developed into an intervention targeting Pacific young people as well as a Pacific leadership programme. *Mana* is an Oceanic word that can be found in 26 Pasifika languages. It refers to power, energy, abundance, authority, miracles – the ability to manifest the energy, flow and fortune of the intangible with grace and efficacy so that it is recognised and impactful in the tangible world. *Moana*, meaning "ocean", is a Polynesian word that can be found in 35 contemporary Pacific languages. *Mana Moana*, then, is about the power, energy and vitality sourced to being from the *moana* and indigenous to the South Pacific region.

Engaging with *Mana Moana* as a body of ancestral knowledge involves a process of decolonisation. It engenders an awakening. It requires socio-historical analysis of how we came to be here, in this position, with this knowledge marginalised. It involves a call to action: a passion for renaissance and reconstruction. It inspires conscious cultural continuity and innovation. Essentially, this is a process of empowering self through authentic engagement with heritage knowledge. It is a process of re-search, re-valuing, re-cognition.

The vision of *Mana Moana* is for Pacific peoples to harness the *mana* and power of who we are and where we are from – to access the knowledge indigenous to the peoples of the waters of the *Moana* – the largest ocean in the world. Our shared linguistic, cultural, genealogical, geographical and historical roots provide us with a treasure trove of rich knowledge that is an essential resource for living wisely and healing today. *Mana Moana* engages generative words, images, metaphors, proverbs and stories.

Words

Mana Moana identifies 70 generative concepts and metaphors found in multiple Pacific languages. Power words are used by groups to communicate about itself, their world, their experiences and their social contexts (Cajete, 1994). Words are considered powerful in our cultures. As they say in Hawaii: *Aia ke ola o ka waha; aia ka make i ka waha*. Life is in the mouth; death is in the mouth – spoken words can enliven and spoken words can destroy (Pukui, Haertig & Lee, 1972). Engaging with these words provides us with alternative resources and ways of narrating stories of self (Garro, 2000) in relationship, connected to the wider world of earth, sea, sky and *atua*, grounded within an ecological perspective that equates healthy relationships with a healthy self. These are words that belong to Pacific peoples collectively and have survived multiple migrations and centuries of linguistic adaptation to remain in at least 15 of our languages today (Greenhill & Clark, 2011).

With *Mana Moana*, the entry into Oceania's library is word by word. Each time we connect to indigenous languages in our present, we connect with the past. Each word is a clue to a whole worldview. The eyes of the ancients and what they once saw is spoken through many of the words engaged with in *Mana Moana*. We focus on and engage with root words, which have been used for centuries in many different Pacific languages to make meaning of the world. The words are Austronesian, Malayo-Polynesian, Oceanic, East Polynesian, Central Polynesian, Fijiac and so on. To engage with them on a deep level is a return and remembering of a common language, of a shared tongue, of a time when we were not so separate.

Images

Many – but not all – of the generative words are illustrated on circular cards and are designed and organised thematically into earth (*fanua/fenua*), sky (*langi*), sea (*moana*), relational spaces between (*va/wa*), family and people (*kainga*) and realm of spirit and archetypal characters and demigods such as Maui (*atua*). As we reflect on the images, the translations, the proverbs, the encircling narratives associated with the words, we ask ourselves two questions about these power words: How do we enhance our regard for it? How do we practice our cognisance of it?

Many of the words – although shared – shift in meaning across the *Moana*. They do not mean exactly the same thing. As they move via migration and survive over centuries of cultural adaption, they may still echo each other but speak in a different tone. The aim is to "open space for multiple ways of interpreting and to invite rather than to define meaning or interpretation" (Tamasese Efi, 2008, p. 71). *Mana Moana* aims to invite meaning, create dialogue, stimulate intergenerational transfer, not define it.

Metaphors

The use of metaphor and figurative language to speak indirectly allows us to "mean more than what we say" (Helu, 1999, p. 60). This maps to a long history of oratory by our leaders and a preferred communication style which is culturally resonant for Pacific peoples (Helu, 1999; Kaeppler, 2002; Mafile'o, 2005; Tamasese Efi, 2003; Taumoepeau, 2004). To draw so heavily on metaphor creates a continuity with cultures that valued oratory, poetry, allusion and indirect ways of communicating. His Highness Tuiatua Tupua Tamasese Ta'isi Efi on pondering our languages noted that it contains deliberate "double-speak" and built in ambivalence – partly to save face – as "loss of face cannot be passed over lightly, loss of face is trauma which inflicts agony persistently and continuously" (Tamasese Efi, 2008, p. 72). In small islands where sustainable relationships are required for peace, collective wellbeing and survival – the use of metaphor, poetry and indirect speech is a way of communicating that maintains relationships even through events of conflict, hostility and stress.

The primary metaphors are embedded within landforms – the library of the land. The *Moana* itself, as well as the shared geographical shapes of shores, reefs, tides, natural life and islands is part of this. These come together to form the structure of this journey. Our landscapes have been deeply theorised by our ancestors, they have storied our worlds and knowledge is encoded into the natural elements. These metaphors gesture to the poetry, artistic sentiment and oratory of our people.

Proverbs

More than 250 proverbs have been collected that reference the generative words. Proverbs in indigenous language from Tongan, Samoan, Niue, Tokelau, Hawaii and Maori that have been translated into English have been collected.

The beauty of proverbs is that they are made to be passed down. They are practical, memorable and bite sized. Proverbs distil and crystallise thinking. They encapsulate values. They are small soundbites of much greater articulations and broader understandings of knowledge. They are perfect for beginners and they do not tire or patronise experts.

In very practical ways, we can harness proverbs into our everyday. We can pass them down to our children. We can use them in our own oratory, both formally and informally. These contextualise the generative concepts in ethnic-specific ways and provide culture-specific nuance and references. They support, scaffold and provide further meaning for generative words and power concepts.

Narratives

Defining narratives and shared stories have been selected which map onto the generative concepts and proverbs. These narratives have emerged from collectivities, expressing deep-rooted cultural themes, passing on narratives of crisis and resolution (Campbell, 1988; Mahina, 1992). When stories are used, as Archibald (2008) points out, the story doesn't tell us what to think or feel, it gives us the space to think and feel (p. 134). Stories contain "narrative resources" that we can use to story our own lives.

By retelling indigenous narratives, we breathe life into ancient resources so that we can ourselves tell better stories about ourselves today. These are not ordinary stories. Our cosmogonies and early "mythology" contain all the seeds and kernels of a cultural world our ancestors created for us over centuries. These are the stories an entire people – including us – live in and through. Revisiting these stories, with respect and love, is to turn a key and unlock a universe that colonisation and Western civilisation has denied us.

The research of our power words and generative concepts, the remembering of these and the recognition that occurs as a part of this work is exciting reconstructive work that helps us make sense of our world today. The search is for ourselves, our language, our knowledge and our stories of the world, which resonates with many, that makes sense, intuitively and fundamentally, to Pacific peoples today.

> **REFLECTION QUESTIONS**
>
> 1. What Pacific-Indigenous concept(s) referenced in this chapter most caught your attention? How has your understanding been extended by the concept(s)?
> 2. What possibilities and challenges do you see in applying Pacific-Indigenous social work theories and models in your practice?

Conclusion

This chapter has provided an introduction to Pacific-Indigenous theories and models for social work practice. The elevation of Pacific knowledge and ways offer an alternative for social work as a whole. A range of examples of how Pacific-Indigenous theories and models may be applied in practice are provided in the fields of practice chapters throughout this book.

References

Archibald, J. (2008). *Indigenous storywork: Educating the heart, mind, body, and spirit.* Vancouver, Canada: UBC Press.

Autagavaia, M. (2001). Social work with Pacific Island Communities. In M. Connolly (Ed.), *New Zealand social work: Contexts and practice.* Melbourne, Australia: Oxford University Press.

Cajete, G. (1994). *Look to the mountain: An ecology of indigenous education.* Durango, CO: Kivaki Press.

Campbell, J. (1988). *The power of myth.* New York: Anchor Books Doubleday.

Child Youth and Family. (2015). *Va'aifetu guardians and guardianship of stars: Principles, cultural frameworks, guidelines.* Wellington, New Zealand: Ministry of Social Development. Retrieved from https://practice.mvcot.govt.nz/documents/knowledge-base-practice-frameworks/working-with-pacific-peoples/vaaifetu-part-2-final.pdf

Coady, N. (2016). The science and art of direct practice: An overview of theory and of a reflective, intuitive-inductive approach to practice. In N. Coady & P. Lehmann (Eds.), *Theoretical perspectives for direct social work practice: A generalist-eclectic approach* (3rd ed., pp. 37–59). New York: Springer.

Crichton-Hill, Y. (2018). Pasifika social work. In M. Connolly, L. Harms & J. Maidment (Eds.), *Social work: Contexts and practice.* Melbourne, Australia: Oxford University Press.

Durie, M. (1985). A Maori perspective of health. *Social Science and Medicine, 20*(5), 483–486.

Durie, M. (2004). Understanding health and illness: Research at the interface between science and indigenous knowledge. *International Journal of Epidemiology, 33*(5), 1138–1143. doi:10.1093/ije/dyh250

Durie, M. (2011). Indigenizing mental health services: New Zealand experience. *Transcultural Psychiatry, 48*(1–2), 24–36.

Faleolo, M. M. (2009). Cultural valid social work education: A Samoan perspective. In C. Noble, M. Henrickson & I. Han (Eds.), *Social work education: Voices from the Asia Pacific* (pp. 149–172). Victoria, Australia: The Vulgar Press.

Garro, L. C. (2000). Cultural knowledge as a resource in illness narratives: Remembering through accounts of illness. In C. G. Mattingly & L. C. Garro (Eds.), *Narrative and the cultural construction of illness and healing* (pp. 70–87). Berkley, CA: University of California Press.

Greenhill, S. & Clark, R. (2011). POLLEX-Online: The Polynesian Lexicon Project Online. *Oceanic Linguistics, 50*(2), 551–559.

Helu, F. (1999). *Critical essays: Cultural perspectives from the South Seas.* Canberra, Australia: The Journal of Pacific History.

Ife, J. (2018). Right-wing populism and social work: Contrasting ambivalences about modernity. *Journal of Human Rights & Social Work, 3*(3), 121.

Johnson, J. T. & Yellow Bird, M. (2012). Indigenous peoples and cultural survival. In L. M. Healy & R. J. Link (Eds.), *Handbook of international social work: Human rights, development, and the global profession* (pp. 208–213). New York: Oxford University Press.

Kaeppler, A. (2002). The structure of Tongan barkcloth design: Imagery, metaphor and allusion. In N. S. A. Herle, K. Stevenson & R. Welsch (Eds.), *Pacific art: Persistence, change and meaning* (pp. 291–308). Honolulu, HI: University of Hawai'i Press.

Mafile'o, T. (2004). Exploring Tongan social work: Fakafekau'aki (connecting) and fakatokilalo (humility). *Qualitative Social Work, 3*(3), 239–257.

Mafile'o, T. (2005). *Tongan metaphors of social work practice: Hangē ha pā kuo fa'u: A thesis presented in partial fulfilment of the requirements for the degree of Doctor of Philosophy in Social Work at Massey University*, Palmerston North, New Zealand: 2005.

Mafile'o, T. (2019, in press). Social work with Pacific communities. In R. Munford & K. O'Donoghue (Eds.), *Emerging theories for social work practice*. London: Jessica Kingsley Publishers.

Mafile'o, T., & Ofahengaue Vakalahi, H. F. (2018). Indigenous social work across borders: Expanding social work in the South Pacific. *International Social Work, 61*(4), 537–552.

Mahina, O. (1992). *The Tongan traditional history tala-ē-fonua: A vernacular ecology-centred historico-cultural concept*. (PhD), Australian National University, Canberra, Australia.

Meo-Sewabu, L. D. (2015). '*Tu ga na inima ka luvu na waqa*': *(The bail to get water out of the boat is in the boat yet the boat sinks): The cultural constructs of health and wellbeing amongst Marama iTaukei in a Fijian village in Lau and in a transnational Fijian community in Whanganui, Aotearoa*. (Social Policy PhD), Massey University, Palmerston North, New Zealand.

Midgley, J. (1981). *Professional imperialism: Social work in the third world*. London: Heinemann.

Mila, K. (2017). Mana Moana: Healing the va, developing spiritually and culturally embedded practices. In L. Béres (Ed.), *Practising spirituality: Reflections on meaning-making in personal and professional contexts* (pp. 61–78). Basingstoke, United Kingdom: Palgrave Macmillan.

Mila-Schaaf, K. (2006). Vā-centred social work: Possibilities for a Pacific approach to social work practice. *Tu Mau/Social Work Review, 18*(1), 8–13.

Ministry of Social Development (2012). *Turanga Māori: A Cook Islands conceptual framework transforming family violence – Restoring wellbeing*. Wellington, New Zealand: Ministry of Social Development.

Mulitalo-Lauta, P. T. (2000). *Fa'asamoa and social work within the New Zealand context*. Palmerston North, New Zealand: Dunmore Press.

Nash, M., O'Donoghue, K. & Munford, R. (2005). *Social work theories in action*. Philadelphia, PA: Jessica Kingsley Publishers.

Newport, C. (2001). Knowing practice Pasifika. *Social Work Review/Tu Mau, 13*(3), 6–9.

Payne, M. (2014). *Modern social work theory* (4th ed.). Basingstoke, United Kingdom: Palgrave Macmillan.

Pukui, M. K., Haertig, E. W. & Lee, C. A. (1972). *Naanaa i ke kumu: Look to the source*. Honolulu, HI: Queen Lili'uokalani Children's Center.

Pulotu-Endemann, K. (2001). *Fonofale model of health*. Pacific Models for Health Promotion. Retrieved from http://apps.centralpho.org.nz/Permalink/MoM/General%20Documents/MoM/Published/Pacific%20Health%20Forms/Fonofale%20model.pdf

Ravulo, J. (2016). Pacific epistemologies in professional social work practice, policy and research. *Asia Pacific Journal of Social Work and Development, 26*(4), 191–202. Doi:10.1080/02185385.2016.1234970

Ravulo, J. (2019, in press). Australian students going to the Pacific Islands: International social work placements and learning across Oceania. *Aotearoa New Zealand Social Work/ Tu Mau*.

Shek, D. T. L., Golightley, M., & Holloway, M. (2017). Editorial: A snapshot of social work in the Asia-Pacific region. *British Journal of Social Work*, 47(1), 1–8. Doi:10.1093/bjsw/bcx007

Tamasese Efi, T. A. T. T. (2003). *In search of meaning, nuance and metaphor in social policy*. Paper presented at the Social Policy Research and Evaluation Conference, Wellington, New Zealand.

Tamasese Efi, T. A. T. T. (2008). *Su'e su'e manogi: In search of fragrance. Tui Atua Tupua Tamasese Ta'isi and the Samoan indigenous reference*. Samoa: Centre for Samoan Studies, National University of Samoa.

Taumoepeau, M. (2004). Ko e heliaki 'i he ngaahi ma'imoa 'a Kuini Salote. In E. Wood-Ellem (Ed.), *Songs and poems of Queen Salote, in English and Tongan* (pp. 104–145). Tonga: Vava'u Press.

Vakalahi, H. F. O., & Godinet, M. T. (2014). *Transnational Pacific Islander Americans and social work: Dancing to the beat of a different drum*. Washington, DC: NASW Press, National Association of Social Workers.

Walter, M. (2013). Geopolitics of sensing and knowing: On (de)coloniality, border thinking, and epistemic disobedience. *Confero: Essays on Education, Philosophy and Politics*, 1(1), 129–150. Doi:10.3384/confero.2001-4562.13v1i1129

Weaver, H. N. (2015). Social work, indigenous ways, and the power of intersection. In C. Fejo-King & P. Mataira (Eds.), *Expanding the conversation: International Indigenous social workers' insights into the use of Indigenist knowledge and theory in practice*. Canberra, Australia: Magpie Goose Publishing.

PART II
Fields of practice

4

SEEING ABILITIES

Disability in the Pacific

Donald Bruce Yeates

Key points

- The rights of people with disabilities in the Pacific are being recognised by Governments at the global and Pacific regional level which cascade through national policies and plans to the local level.
- The experiences of Pacific people with disabilities at the local level indicate that people face disability-discrimination barriers that prevent their realising their full potential and participation in family/living groups and community affairs.
- Partnering with people with disabilities to narrate their personal experiences creates understanding and enables individuals to be fully integrated into families/living groups and communities and the realisation of their rights.

Introduction

A broken left ankle with a cast and on crutches, I was standing at the bottom of the stairs leading up to the classroom at the University of Papua New Guinea. There was a dilemma – I had a lecture to give in five minutes time, stairs to mount, on crutches, having just learned how to use them on flat surfaces and holding a bag with teaching materials. One of my students who had been physically disabled since early childhood walked past me on her crutch, said hello, nimbly climbed the stairs and looked back at me with a smile on her face and proceeded on to the classroom to await my arrival and the start of the lecture.

> **REFLECTION**
>
> Three observations from this personal experience:
>
> 1. Disability can be long term or short term and can occur at any age no matter what one's gender or social economic status.
> 2. Societal structures and attitudes pose barriers for disabled people preventing full participation in one's family/living group, community and society at large.
> 3. Society is prone to overlook one's abilities.

People with disabilities in the Pacific demonstrate strength and resilience as evidenced in the ability to transcend societal barriers and disability-based discrimination that have denied persons with disabilities equitable access to education, employment, housing and public services. People with disabilities have been excluded from family and community life, often living in poverty, as manifest in its many forms, and on the margins of society.

The 2011 *World Report on Disability* defines disability as

> an umbrella term for impairments, activity limitations, and participation restrictions. Disability refers to the negative aspects of the interaction between individuals with a health condition (such as cerebral palsy, Down syndrome, depression) and personal and environmental factors (such as negative attitudes, inaccessible transportation and public buildings, and limited social supports).
>
> *(World Health Organisation, 2011)*

Article 1 of The United Nations *Convention on the Rights of the Persons with Disabilities* (CRPD) specifies that "[p]ersons with disabilities include those who have long-term physical, mental, intellectual or sensory impairments which in interaction with various barriers may hinder their full and effective participation in society on an equal basis with others" (United Nations, 2006).

The Pacific Disability Forum estimated that there were 1.708 million people with disabilities living in the Pacific (Pacific Disability Forum, 2018a). Ageing (World Health Organisation, 2011), non-communicable diseases, natural and human disasters, diet and substance abuse, health issues arising from fallout of nuclear testing on Pacific atolls and islands are examples of health and environmental factors that account for these numbers.

Global and Pacific regional statistics can be daunting for practitioners and practice skills are needed to disaggregate this data and make sense of it for the national and local context. National population censuses and household surveys can aid one in this task. Surveys undertaken by consultants working for international development partners and regional and national associations "for and of" disabled persons provide both quantitative and qualitative data informing one's practice. A good example is *A Deeper Silence: The Unheard Experiences of Women with Disabilities and Their Sexual and Reproductive Health Experiences: Kiribati, the Solomon Islands and Tonga* (Spratt, 2012).

From the title of the report itself, one can immediately discern that the information and data are disaggregated by sex – women; barrier – silence and unheard; health issue – sexual and reproductive health;[1] country contexts – Kiribati, Solomon Islands and Tonga. For each country, we see that a situation analysis has been completed and information has been provided on disability in general, the legislation and services provided for people with disabilities, the personal experiences of women with disabilities and recommendations for action and practice. This information adds value to one's understanding of disability in the specified countries and also for social and community workers in other countries who may be working with people with disabilities who come from Kiribati, Solomon Islands or Tonga.

A key feature of the local qualitative information from *A Deeper Silence* is the "unheard experiences" of the women with disabilities. Statistical data can give one the number and types of disabilities and locate where people with disabilities reside – but social and community workers need to hear and listen to the stories of disabled people with whom they work. Through learning and listening to the story, one is validating the personal experience, connecting people to others and giving agency to the individual in the context of their family/living group and community (Tascón, 2018; see also Bell, 2017; Tofuaipangai, 2016).

Disability in the Pacific: Global convention, regional framework and national policy[2]

The United Nations Convention on the Rights of Persons with Disabilities (CRPD) had been ratified by 13 Pacific Island countries[3] (including Australia and New Zealand) and 2 countries[4] had signed the Convention. In ratifying the Convention, countries are legally bound to implement the terms of the Convention in their respective jurisdictions while those countries that have only signed the Convention must refrain from impeding or working against the terms and conditions of the Convention (Pacific Disability Forum, 2018a). Ratification means that social workers are obligated to ensure that the terms and conditions of the Convention are integrated into relevant country legislation, ensure that appropriate policies are in place for government, private sector and civil society organisations and act as disability rights advocates in their practice. Ratification also implies a shift in power relations within organisations and between practitioners and people with disabilities – from "control and doing things for" to "partnership and working with".

The Pacific Framework for the Rights of Persons with Disabilities (PFRPD) 2016–2025 provides Pacific governments and other organisations a means of implementing the articles of the Convention on the Rights of Persons with Disabilities (Pacific Islands Forum Secretariat, 2016). The strategies outlined in the Framework are geared toward the organisational members of the Council of Regional Organisations of the Pacific (CROP),[5] UN entities based in the Pacific, private sector and Pacific regional non-government and faith-based organisations.

By its nature, the Framework is a managerial, top-down oriented and largely externally funded set of strategies. The Framework was developed through the consultative and decision-making processes of the Pacific Islands Forum in collaboration with the Pacific Disability Forum. The Framework aims for inclusive development and is structured around five main goals – Livelihoods, Mainstreaming, Leadership and Enabling Environment, Disaster Risk Management and Evidence.[6] The document aligns Pacific regional disability initiatives with the Convention on the Rights of Persons with Disabilities, the Sustainable Development Goals (SDG),[7] and the Incheon Strategy.[8] The Framework's second goal, "Mainstreaming", stipulates strategies and outcomes that will ensure that national, local and community policies are inclusive of the rights of persons with disabilities and also will ensure that participation and meeting the needs of women with disabilities are explicitly identified.

A 2012 Mapping Report found that there were approved or draft national disability policies and plans in most countries surveyed but that implementation was "overall weak given that in all countries there is none or a minimal budget allocation by government to disability programs" (Pacific Disability Forum, 2012). This finding is a national disability discrimination barrier in its own right. While Pacific governments are systematically developing appropriate policies and plans, the key to effective policy implementation lies in the annual national budget allocations. Social workers need to know the annual national budget process, locate national ministries responsible for disability and lobby for national budget allocations for disability programmes across ministries.

CROP agencies such as The University of the South Pacific (USP) provide resources for inclusive development at the national level. USP is owned by 12 member governments[9] and has 14 campuses across the Pacific region. The USP has a Disability Inclusiveness Policy (The University of the South Pacific, 2013) and its Disability Resource Centre[10] is responsible for providing disability support services to students and staff across the campuses of the University. Hearing and learning from USP students with disabilities such as Leslie Tikotikoca is one way of inspiring young disabled people and their families to seek opportunities for higher education in the Pacific.

> **CASE STUDY 4.1: LESLIE**
>
> Leslie was 13 years old when he stepped on a live power line. He was hospitalised for four months in Suva and New Zealand. He lost his leg, had to learn to speak and had to re-gain the use of his left hand. All through this period he had the support of his parents and siblings. Leslie was able to stand before the new students at the official USP Orientation Welcome Day, and confidently say "I am a human with a lot of abilities and talents and I love to live life" (Mala, 2017).

Pacific social workers engaged at the family and community level will have to work using local, national and regional financial, physical and human resources to effect inclusive development.

Pacific social work practice and models

Pacific social work practice uses a "rights based approach" when informed by the Convention on the Rights of Persons with Disabilities and the Pacific Framework for the Rights of Persons with Disabilities. These global and regional documents emphasise the universal values of human rights and social justice, which through inter-organisational consultation cascade into national disability policies and plans. In using a rights-based approach, social workers are also called upon to "recognize and respect the inherent dignity and worth of all human beings in attitude, word, and deed" (International Federation of Social Workers, 2018). The implementation of these values at the local level must be negotiated into specific cultural contexts and address the needs of people with disabilities in their families and communities. Social workers in this scenario "have to think and act globally and locally, holding the global and the local in tension, but making it a creative tension" (Ife, 2018).

The tensions that arise for the practitioner are often the result of a clash between world views. At the local level, the social worker's world view starts with the experience of the "particular" – the experience of "this" person with a disability, the experience of "this" family, the experience of "this" community and works towards the global universals. The rights-based approach starts with the universal values and tries to fit people with disabilities into a universal belief system, managed through specific strategies and measured by outcomes – the result often being the experiences of the particular reduced to statistics.

Social workers need to frame rights-based practice in the local cultural context (top-down practice) and in turn inform the implementation process through the lens of local norms and values of the particular experiences of persons with disabilities (bottom-up practice). And these experiences are often communicated through stories and other forms of artistic expression (Tascón, 2018).

Nai Dabedabe and *Mango tree*

Nai Dabedabe and *Mango Tree* are two examples of Pacific epistemologies (or ways of knowing). They were developed by social workers in Fiji who were challenged to develop models of social work practice that respected "their own cultural worldviews and those of their clients" (Lal, 2005, p. 14).

The image of *Nai Dabedabe* (Fijian seat or stool) has been used as a model of practice in Fiji (Nainoca, 2005). The raised top of the four legged stool focuses attention on the client supported by the four legs: *Na Lotu* – church, spirituality, religion; *Nai Tavi* – employment, responsibility and obligation; *Na Vuli* – education and training; and *Na Vuvale* – the family in all its forms. The braces and binding are seen as the social worker holding the supports in position utilising the practice skills and facilitating meeting the needs of the client. When applying the model in the local context one needs to be specific of the particular – this person with a disability living in this family and/or living group, in this community. *Na Lotu* implies the network of civil society faith-based and non-government organisations. In a village there can be an array of both internal and external organisations competing for the "disability space" and social workers need to work with the "client" on which one or ones best meet their needs. *Nai Tavi* focuses on the physical employment or vocation of the person with a disability. What are their aspirations? How best can these be met? What support is needed in order to achieve these? *Na Vuli* refers to the education and training needed by the person both to achieve their employment aspirations and to participate fully in family and community life. *Na Vuvale* – the family has culturally been the basic social unit and foundation for the care, wellbeing and identity of the individual. People with disabilities have been cared for by the extended family unit and in some instances have been kept separate from community living through caring over-protection, which prevents the person from developing to their full potential (Sera, 2018). *Nai Vakasaia* is the social worker's counsel provided to the individuals concerned. Through meaningful *talanoa*,[11] the social worker is able to engage with families on how various needs may be met utilising local and regional resources.

The *Mango Tree* has been used in Fiji to convey *zindagi ka safar* (the journey of life) and the tree's parts are symbolic of human development through the life span, as the individual person with a disability negotiates their world view in the context of the family and community (Lal, 2005). The parts of the mango tree has many uses as does a disabled person have many abilities – from the preserves made from the green mango, the eating of the ripe fruit, the leaf for healing and prayer to the bark used for medicinal purposes. The mangoes are sold in the market. The strong roots support the tree as does the good nurturing of children in diverse family backgrounds. The trunk represents the knowledge gained and used by individuals as they interact with the world around them. Inter-personal family and community relationships are represented through the branches. The branches also denote the societal network of support services and protection. The leaves provide shelter and shade as does the family support the individual.

The blooming flowers signify that one is ready to have a family. The fruit signifies the fullness of one's life and the seed of the fruit reproduction and new life – the right of people with disabilities to have a full rewarding life, to have children and to have healthy sexual relationships.

Nai Dabedabe and the *Mango Tree* generic models of Pacific social work practice share a common set of values and norms that emphasise the collective, communal nature of family and community relationships. Setareki Macanawai sums this value up in the indigenous concept of *Vanua* – "Vanua is a traditional, indigenous concept embracing people and the land. It is how we in Fiji, and in much of the Pacific Islands, respect our land, our culture, and our values. It is about sharing and caring for the collective" (Sera, 2018, para. 1). Practitioners must embed this value but not sentimentalise it. Ipul Powaseu points out that traditionally in Papua New Guinea caring for the needy was a cultural norm based on a communal system. The value of caring has eroded and negatively affects people with disabilities, with many having to be on the streets of the main urban centres – selling items to support themselves and their families (Powaseu, 2009). Social workers need to embrace the particular experience and assist in the narration of that experience to the wider community.

PRACTICE EXAMPLE 4.1

When I was young I got sick and it affected the growth of my leg. I had to learn to walk with a crutch and was left out of many things in the life of the village. I felt different to all the other children. I had negative feelings about my life because of the way I was treated. My mother treated me well and protected me. The Catholic sisters at the school encouraged my parents to let me go to school. Eventually they did even though I was a girl and had a disability.

REFLECTIVE QUESTIONS

1. What is this story telling you about people with disabilities?
2. How could you use this story in your social work practice?

Source: Author's construct based on experience and relevant literature.

Conclusion

"Recognition to Realisation of Rights" (Pacific Disability Forum, 2018b) reflects the state of play about disability in the Pacific. Governments have ratified or signed the Convention on the Rights of Persons with Disabilities, endorsed the Pacific Framework for the Rights of Persons with Disabilities and have developed national disability policies and plans. Strategic partnerships have been established between organisations for and of the disabled which are taking actions to achieve the aims of the Framework and mainstream the rights of the persons with disabilities in the broader legislation and policies of respective governments. Social workers are called upon to be disability rights' advocates and through their ethical practice to recognise the inherent dignity of humanity. Social workers need to work globally and locally, framing these universal rights and ethical principles in the context of local culture, values and norms. The rights-based approach may lead to recognition of the rights of persons with disabilities at the national level and to some extent the family and community level. It is the particular experiences of people with disabilities that need to be heard and narrated, creating understanding, enabling individuals to be fully integrated into families/living groups and communities and the realisation of their rights.

Notes

1. See Chapter 12: An introduction to sexual and reproductive health and wellbeing for Pacific social workers.
2. For a fuller discussion on the relationship between social policy and practice see Chapter 18: Navigating social policy processes in the Pacific.
3. Countries that had ratified the CRPD as of 2017: Australia, Cook Islands, Federated States of Micronesia, Fiji, Kiribati, Nauru, New Zealand, Palau, Papua New Guinea, Republic of the Marshall Islands, Samoa, Tuvalu, Vanuatu.
4. Countries that had signed but not ratified the CRPD as of 2017: Solomon Islands and Tonga.
5. CROP agencies include: Secretariat of the Pacific Community (SPC) (formerly the South Pacific Commission),
Forum Fisheries Agency (FFA), South Pacific Regional Environment Program (SPREP), Pacific Islands Development Program (PIDP), South Pacific Travel Organisation (SPTO), The University of the South Pacific (USP), Pacific Aviation Safety Organisation and Pacific Power Association. The Pacific Islands Forum Secretariat acts as CROP's permanent chair and provides secretariat support (Australian Government, 2018).
6. See Chapter 7: Pacific-Indigenous community-village resilience in disasters.
7. The United Nations 2030 Agenda for Sustainable Development and its 17 Sustainable Development Goals adopted by world leaders at the UN Summit in 2015. The SDG succeeded the Millennium Development Goals (MDG) 2000–2015.
8. The ESCAP Incheon Strategy is the Asia-Pacific 2013–2022 regionally agreed disability-inclusive development goals.
9. USP member countries: Cook Islands, Fiji, Kiribati, Marshall Islands, Nauru, Niue, Samoa, Solomon Islands, Tokelau, Tonga, Tuvalu and Vanuatu.
10. USP received accreditation by the WASC Senior College and University Commission (WSCUC) based in California, United States of America. WSCUC commended the University for meeting the core competencies and standards among which was the eighth commendation: "The Disability Resource Centre that provides support and accommodations, and fosters a strong community, continuing to expand accessibility for students with disabilities throughout the region" (Studley, 2018).

11 "Talanoa is a generic term referring to a conversation, chat, sharing of ideas and talking with someone. ... shared by Tongans, Samoans, and Fijians. Talanoa is used ... to teach a skill, to share ideas, ... to resolve problems, to build and maintain relationships" (Johansson Fua, 2018).

References

Australian Government. (2018, September 14). *Department of Foreign Affairs and Trade*. Retrieved from https://dfat.gov.au/international-relations/regional-architecture/pacific-islands/Pages/council-of-regional-organisations-in-the-pacific-crop.aspx

Bell, H. A. (2017, March 14). Introducing the special issue: Social work and the narrative (half?) turn. *Qualitative Social Work*, *16*(2), 161–165.

Ife, J. (2018, September 6). Decolonising community development for global practice. *Presentation at the Mini-Symposium – Niu Directions Across Oceania: Implications for Social & Community Development Practice*. Suva, Fiji: School of Social Sciences, The University of the South Pacific.

International Federation of Social Workers. (2018, July 2). *Global Social Work Statement of Ethical Principles*. Retrieved from www.ifsw.org/global-social-work-statement-of-ethical-principles/

Johansson Fua, S. (2018, October 1). *Kakala Research Framework*. Retrieved from http://repository.usp.ac.fj/8197/1/Kakala_Research_Framework_Seuula_Johansson-Fua.pdf

Lal, J. D. (2005, November). Zindagi Ka Safar – Mango tree framework. *The Fiji Social Workers Journal*, *1*(1), 3–16.

Mala, S. (2017, January 31). *Student In Crutches Overcomes Hurdles*. Retrieved from http://fijisun.com.fj/2017/01/31/student-in-crutches-overcomes-hurdles/

Nainoca, M. G. (2005, November). Nai Dabedabe: A model of practice for social work in Fiji. *The Fiji Social Workers Journal*, *1*, 8–11.

Pacific Disability Forum. (2012). *Mapping of the disability policy and program frameworks in the Pacific*. Suva, Fiji: Government of Australia, AusAid.

Pacific Disability Forum. (2018a, September 4). *Pacific Disability Forum*. Retrieved from www.pacificdisability.org/About-Us/Disability-in-the-Pacific.aspx

Pacific Disability Forum. (2018b, May 9). *PDF – 6TH Pacific Regional Conference on Disability*. Retrieved from www.pacificdisability.org/Home/PDF-6TH-Pacific-Regional-Conference-on-Disability.aspx

Pacific Islands Forum Secretariat. (2016). *Pacific framework for the rights of persons with disabilities 2016–2025*. Suva, Fiji: Pacific Islands Forum Secretariat.

Powaseu, I. (2009, October 14). *Stand Up Against Poverty*. Retrieved from www.onejustworld.com.au/forums/Stand-Up-Against-Poverty?Speaker=Ipul-Powaseu

Sera, Y. W. (2018, August 8). *Indigenous Concept of Vanua: Empowering Indigenous Persons with Disabilities*. Retrieved from https://internationalfunders.org/indigenous-concept-of-vanua-empowering-indigenous-persons-with-disabilities/

Spratt, J. M. (2012). *A deeper silence: The unheard experiences of women with disabilities and their sexual and reproductive health experiences: Kiribati, the Solomon Islands and Tonga*. Suva, Fiji: United Nations Population Fund Pacific Sub-Regional Office.

Studley, J. S. (2018, September 18). *Commission Action Letter, Seeking Accreditation Visit 1, June 2018 Action*. Retrieved from www.usp.ac.fj/index.php?id=22504

Tascón, S. M. (2018, September 6). Digital story telling for social work practice. *Presentation at the Mini- Symposium – Nui Directions Across Oceania: Implications for Social and Community Work Practice*. Suva, Fiji: School of Social Sciences, The University of the South Pacific.

The University of the South Pacific. (2013, April 10). *Disability Inclusiveness Policy*. Retrieved from https://policylib.usp.ac.fj/

Tofuaipangai, S. C. (2016). Social policy, social work and fatongia: Implications of the Tongan concept of obligation. *Aotearoa New Zealand Social Work, 28*(1), 60–67.

United Nations. (2006). *United Nations Convention on the Rights of Persons with Disabilities*. United Nations.

World Health Organisation. (2011). *World Report on Disability*. World Health Organisation.

5
UNDERSTANDING MENTAL HEALTH AND WELLBEING FROM A PACIFIC PERSPECTIVE

Jioji Ravulo, Monique Faleafa and Tanya Koro

Key points
- Ensuring Pacific perspectives are included in the context in which mental health issues are understood is key to developing mental health literacies and knowledge across Pacific communities.
- Promoting psycho-education to family members who are striving to effectively support their relative with a mental illness can help recovery.
- Indigenous knowledges and practice approaches are also vital to ensuring contemporary service provision and delivery are inclusive of cultural values and views.

Pacific people and mental health

Mental health is a burgeoning field of research and practice in and across society. The way in which mental health has been captured to include the notion of mental health illnesses or issues has also been a relatively new area that social workers and other allied health professionals have focused on. That is, traditionally, mental health was seen as being imbedded into western medical models of health alone, and not fully understood and appreciated from a holistic view of wellbeing. With this new focus comes a new array of perspectives and approaches, with many new ways developed within a westernised frame of thinking. However, despite the separation and greater nuancing of mental health illnesses across society, there are certain differences that may exist in and across Pacific communities. This includes an evolving understanding of mental health and wellbeing as a concept within traditional views that permeate Pacific culture. This chapter will explore the various differences that may exist in the way in which mental health and wellbeing is perceived by Pacific people, whilst also reviewing possible opportunities and strategies to effectively engage in developing new and contemporary perspectives amongst Pacific communities.

Social work perspectives around mental health and wellbeing (macro/meso/micro)

Within a social work framework, mental health issues can be seen within a bio-psycho-social approach "that addresses the physical, psychological and social aspects of the client and their situation, including meeting basic needs, family interactions, significant relationships, social support and cultural factors" (Connolly, Harms & Maidment, 2018, p. 306). From this view, the need to ensure that mental health assessments are carried out through a holistic manner that truly incorporates this approach in practice is an important part of being able to then create possible solutions and strategies to support wellbeing. However, this can be greatly challenged by competing priorities for social workers across the various areas in which they may carry out work related to mental health and wellbeing, deterring a greater opportunity to deal appropriately and adequately with such a need. This includes the lack of consistent funding to employ suitably qualified and trained practitioners in fields within statutory health and community settings, paired with a lack of understanding and appreciation for the need to carry out such work across the local community. With more research being undertaken in this field of practice over the last decade (Ataera-Minster & Trowland, 2018), it has improved the political will from governments across Oceania, including Australia, New Zealand and Pacific Islands countries to see their role in supporting a health sector needing to be ever responsive to such issues. The increase in mental health services for young people has improved in various spaces, and the resource base is changing. In some countries where there is a large Pacific diaspora like New Zealand, specific Pacific-related resources have improved, however, in other areas like Australia, Pacific or Indigenous specificity in the role of mental health and wellbeing is still lacking.

Other key social work perspectives also striving to assist in challenging the way in which society views mental health and wellbeing includes the anti-oppressive approach, where issues are exacerbated through structural, cultural and personal levels of oppression. The need to challenge the way in which society as a whole views mental health illness will create a greater opportunity for a cultural shift to occur, where people may be encouraged to acknowledge the true impacts on an individual, and where personal mental health issues are provided with the ability to seek appropriate support for recovery. From a broader societal viewpoint, it may be evident within a Western context that changes are occurring at the structural level where governments are now funding institutions to be better equipped to promote recovery, in turn creating a culture across society where people are raising the need to access support, which enables individuals to seek and gain support. However, from a Pacific perspective, this uptake of services for individuals may be deterred by a lack of understanding within traditional cultural perspectives on mental health and wellbeing within a medical/health framework, which in turn deters a lack of political will and understanding at the government/structural/institutional level to do something adequate to enact change in this area.

Therefore, part of the solution in creating a greater understanding and uptake of mental health service delivery and provision within Pacific people across Oceania, including those in the diaspora, may rely on more than the understanding of the bio-psycho-social and anti-oppressive approach. Rather, a collective and shared approach in creating new research, policy and practice perspectives that will support such development in this field of practice across the region is needed.

Understanding Pacific mental health research

In 2017, Le Va, a mental health organisation in New Zealand, established to enhance the quality of services to Pacific people and grow the Pacific workforce, published *Kato Fetu: Review of the Pacific Mental Health and Addiction Research Agenda*. The report highlights five priority areas needing to be further explored in the hope of promoting an inclusive conversation around appropriate assessment, intervention or treatment for Pacific people by understanding mental health and addiction, enhancing service responsiveness, developing the workforce, including Pacific people with experience of mental illness and promoting Pacific child and adolescent mental health (Le Va, 2017). It is envisioned that through these key priority areas, a holistic approach is adopted where strategies, structures and systems are meaningfully created alongside resources to holistically deal with the issues associated with mental health and wellbeing.

As western societies tend to create services that are catered for individual views and responses, the need to promote services that include the bigger picture of the individual and their context, including significant others and their impact on wellbeing, is vital. This involves ensuring assessment tools are utilised that capture information from the family, peer and community context hence promoting a micro, meso and macro perspective often found in the anti-oppressive approach used in social work. Exploring the individuals' context and response to how they interact with personal, cultural and structural factors may greatly assist the way in which intervention strategies are employed to help make a genuine difference. The way in which a family may effectively respond to a fellow family member having a mental health illness, and the support they may provide in ensuring adequate assistance is given, can help implement positive recovery.

In essence, such a holistic response within a Pacific context is normal from a traditional and cultural view, as our sense of individuality is inextricably bound and connected to the self and others. The need to cater for other's wellbeing is embedded in our shared consciousness that we live not just to support our own wellbeing, but the wellbeing of others in and around the space in which we occupy. This concept of space is captured by the notion of *Vā* (Mila-Schaaf, 2006;

Mila-Schaaf & Hudson, 2009), which ensures people are in the right relationship with each other in and across families and communities. Being able to support the recovery of a Pacific person who experiences mental health issues may include ensuring a supportive, caring relationship with the self and others, and bringing balance by nurturing *Vā*. This includes enhancing a genuine connection to space and place, and reiterating a bigger purpose and association – beyond the isolation that mental illnesses may bring to an individual.

Therefore, the need to create resources and practice approaches that are nuanced and influenced by Pacific perspectives is well supported by the literature in the context of mental health and wellbeing. For young people, research suggests being able to promote the use of "community organising" by Pacific youth for Pacific youth which can provide scope for agency, and the development of a broader conversation associated with such issues (Han et al., 2015). We need to help promote a shared conversation about such need across the community – empowering the community to have their voices profiled, heard, understood and meaningfully incorporated into our bourgeoning definition of mental health and wellbeing across our community. Pacific people need to be given the platform to contribute to such conversations, and this example provides a starting point for this. Being strategic in the development of Pacific inclusion across various levels to support the meaningful presence of such voices is important (Smith & Jury, 2017). Organisations like Le Va in New Zealand, who are also working on projects supporting other countries across Oceania, is an example that promotes the development of a skilled workforce that exercises culturally aware and appropriate ways to enhance the uptake of Pacific people in mental health service delivery and provision. This of course relies heavily on governance structures being receptive to such issues and needs. Hence, across the broader region, having more Pacific people partnered with such organisations can support the prevalence of such work and the scope to enact change.

Need for broader mental health policies across Oceania

Various governments across the broader Pacific region are developing their own strategies on counteracting the disease burden of mental illness across their community. The establishment of the Vanuatu Mental Health Policy and Strategic Plan (Vanuatu Ministry of Health, 2016) provides a promising framing to creating long term solutions, but it still requires traditional perspectives to meaningfully pervade the way in which cultural values and expectations are included in making a positive impact. From a western perspective, it provides a good overarching strategy on the need to create key signposts and outcomes in mental health, however, it still needs to meaningfully ensure local people are part of this process of meeting such goals.

This also includes the various actions being considered by key regional bodies like the Pacific Community (also known as SPC – Secretariat of the Pacific Community) who are actively involved as per their website "in being able to bring a multi-disciplinary approach to addressing some of the region's most complex development challenges, including climate change, disasters, non-communicable diseases, gender equality, youth employment, food and water security, and biosecurity for trade" (Pacific Community, 2018). Working also in accordance with the United Nations Sustainable Development Goals (SDGs), each member state is committed to promoting regional collaboration, whilst strengthening and enhancing expertise and knowledge through planning and evaluation alongside appropriate systems. However, despite SPC's strategic goal to support public health systems and approaches, there is no specific mention of mental health and wellbeing in their 2016–2020 strategic plan (Pacific Community, 2015). Unfortunately, with competing demands across the region, a lack of focus on mental health in this high-level policy space can limit prioritisation of mental health policy and its implementation for small island nations. It can impact on the way in which governance structures adequately plan and integrate mental health policies for Pacific people, which would in turn support other legislative development to adequately fund resources in government budgets. Therefore, the need to be more mindful, especially as social workers strive to make a contribution to areas of policy for good mental health and wellbeing, is still an ongoing process across Oceania, including countries like Australia and New Zealand, who are also part of the work undertaken by SPC. Nonetheless, it is pleasing to see the United Nations Sustainable Development Goals now inclusive of the notion of mental health and wellbeing, specifically in SDG #3, and the importance this places on nations employing these goals to include such strategies in their planning and processes.

Despite this lack of strategic purpose at the regional level around responsive policy, there are ground swells of activity occurring in various Pacific Islands, including Tonga. During Mental Health Week in 2017, a group of proactive health and education professionals hosted the first ever mental health conference to further highlight the need to promote adequate services (Tonga National Health and Disabilities Association, 2017). Under the key theme of "Understanding the place and state of mental health in Tonga" the five-day symposium strove to further profile the need to start ongoing conversations to bolster the way in which mental health is understood beyond the spiritual to also the medical and health context. It is within such localised movements that further conversations may occur, but it does require the ongoing dedication and time from local Pacific champions to sustain such vision and voices to ensure Pacific people are given the opportunity to participate in appropriate support and assistance.

Social work practice made Pacific

From an individual level, it is important to position the initial case management or counselling assessment process to include a broader family perspective. By using social work approaches intertwined with Pacific perspectives like *talanoa* (Vaka, Brannelly & Huntington, 2016) and *Vā* whilst also incorporating a family systems approach, practitioners are able to gain a greater insight into the roles and responsibilities played out by individuals that make up a family. Be mindful though that the notion of a "nuclear" family is not generally fixed in Pacific communities, as extended family members are also part of a much broader and bigger system that makes up the notion of family. This may include a significant contribution of grandparents, aunts and uncles, cousins and other key peers that may be based on kinship ties and regional relationships forged by village connections and contributions. Practically, the use of a genogram can be a helpful way to work with an individual to gain insight into who makes up their family, past and present, whilst also exploring the type of relationships and dynamics that occurs within that family system.

In supporting the individual work towards effective intervention and support in recovery, it is also important to gain genuine involvement from family members. The role of psychoeducation through the *talanoa* approach – where significant people involved in the individual's life receives accessible information on how to support their loved one – is also part of this process. Accessing existing material made available via reputable online resources and professional services that are providing support can assist in having a positive conversation with such people around how they can best understand and proactively support the needs of their loved one in their recovery. Information on symptoms, how they manifest in behaviours, the impacts and effects of medications and where to get further support is also part of psychoeducation and can help combat any negative stigma surrounding mental illness. The use of online resources can provide a greater platform for support, but it still needs to be provided in a manner that is inclusive of cultural differences including those based on socio-economic status, language and ability (Social Policy Evaluation and Research Unit, 2016). Being able to ensure young people and their support have the scope to access such online websites and phone-based applications does rely heavily on internet availability, which may be limited to some individuals and families. However, supporting youth and adults to access spaces that have such technology, like local schools, libraries and community centres, can also provide an opportunity for face to face services including counselling support, or other forms of information, support and services to be provided.

From a broader perspective, increasing mental health literacies within Pacific communities across the region will also assist with addressing stigma and the morbidity of an undiagnosed or untreated mental health issue. As previously mentioned, a common worldview of having a mental illness in the Pacific is perceived as being either a spiritual issue or an ability to inadequately deal with the self and others – to deal with disruption in the *Vā* held between people, the environment or ancestors. There is a dire need to develop relevant resources that address mental health issues from this holistic perspective of wellbeing. Informative pamphlets and digital resources are a good start, but education at grass roots level involving co-design for local solutions is the gold-standard practice required to truly address mental wellbeing in Pacific populations.

Understanding mental health and wellbeing 53

CASE STUDY 5.1: ANA

Background history

Ana is a 14-year-old Tongan student living at home with her parents and five siblings. Ana is the youngest child and only daughter of the parents. Ana's parents both work full time and her father and older brothers own a small company. Ana was temporarily placed in the care of her grandfather three years prior to presenting to secondary mental health due to reported physical abuse in the home.

The School Counsellor, Stella, reports Ana is a good student with aspirations of becoming a civil engineer. However, Ana was beginning to miss school and disengaged from her peers, which led to a referral from her Form Teacher to the School Counsellor. Ana has built a good rapport with Stella and has been seeing her for five weeks prior to this urgent referral to the secondary mental health team. Ana disclosed historical sexual assault by a church member at the age of ten. Ana's best friend Laura lives next door and is the only person apart from the counsellor who is aware of the effect the trauma is having on her.

Client's situation

Ana reported active suicidal ideation to the counsellor for two weeks, which developed into suicide intent. Ana disclosed to the counsellor that she planned to kill herself in her room and was in the process of doing so when her friend Laura walked into the room. Laura stopped her and pleaded with Ana to tell her parents or talk to someone; hence the disclosure to the school counsellor. Stella contacted the secondary mental health service out of concern for Ana's safety. Stella requested an urgent appointment on the same day as she feared Ana would attempt again if she went home.

The mental health team accepted the request and an appointment was scheduled for 3pm on the same day. Ana presented at the Mental Health Service with the support of Stella. Ana and Stella were initially greeted by two mental health clinicians upon arrival. Stella insisted that she take the lead disclosing her concerns to Ana's parents.

The counsellor contacted Ana's parents requesting their presence at the appointment. Ana's parents were not aware their daughter was seeing the school counsellor, that she reported historic sexual assault and was actively suicidal. Ana's father was accompanied to the appointment by her two older brothers and their mother arrived soon afterwards.

Stella was in the process of explaining her concerns and the reason/s for requesting an urgent mental health assessment to the clinicians when Ana's parents arrived. Ana's parents were distraught when they arrived at the Mental Health Service, they were confused as to why their daughter was at a mental health facility with a stranger. Introductions were led by one of the clinicians, including names and specific roles. The parent's confusion and distress escalated to anger and frustration after Stella gave a brief summary regarding the circumstances which led to this appointment. Stella reported her concerns around Ana's safety, the suicide attempts and the reported historical sexual assault. The situation escalated to raised voices, tears from both Ana and her mother and the father trying to calm his sons from yelling at Ana to give them the name of the perpetrator.

Ana's mother was extremely angry with Stella for withholding information about her daughter's wellbeing from her, for not contacting them regarding Ana's reported suicide attempt in the first instance and for being culturally insensitive and disrespectful around the way she reported the above to them. The mental health team apologised to Ana's parents for the way they were informed and provided some context on Stella's obligations to maintaining confidentiality if this was requested by Ana under the Privacy Act.

A formal mental health assessment was conducted with Ana reporting poor sleep patterns, lowered mood, loss of interest in activities she would usually enjoy, low appetite, isolating herself from friends at school except for her best friend next door, feeling worthless and intermittent suicidal thoughts and intent.

Support given

Talanoa sessions with trained mental health clinicians were conducted with both Ana and her mother, as well as separate individual therapy sessions for Ana. Psychoeducation was provided for Ana's parents and brothers around the impact of trauma on mental health and wellbeing. Removing guilt, shame and the need for parents to reposition their blaming on themselves was also addressed. Psychoeducation was also provided for Ana using the *Fonofale* model of health and wellbeing, where she identified internal strengths and abilities alongside her family, school and broader community networks for ongoing support and assistance.

Outcomes

Ana was prescribed naturally derived herbal sleep drops due to her parents not supporting psychiatric medication for their daughter. Her parents reinstated family *talanoa* processes in their home with the children giving each other the space and opportunity to discuss their dreams, concerns and wellbeing with each other. They scheduled "coffee dates" with Ana to nurture the relationship with her. Her parents are also now attending workshops with other Pasifika families in the community to share and receive ideas on how to better support Ana and her siblings.

Reflection on providing support to Ana within a Pacific context

Engaging the wider family support system by including a culturally relevant *Talanoa* approach with Ana's treatment and psychoeducation was key for her recovery. Carefully integrating cultural processes such as *Talanoa* with a bio-psycho-social assessment and treatment approach was beneficial for Ana and her parents and siblings.

Overall, this case study highlights some crucial elements to consider and reflect upon as social workers:

- The need to have a broader awareness and understanding of existing structures, what is considered *tabu* and the role of sacred relationships including the concepts of *Vā* within Pacific families and communities.
- An importance to acknowledge and negotiate the existing tension between maintaining confidentiality on behalf of young Pacific service users whilst building initial and ongoing rapport with their parents and families.
- Ensuring Pacific young people with mental health issues are fully informed around the advantages and disadvantages of sharing information with their parents and families. Whilst informed consent is necessary, when working with young people, "informed assent" may be sought by the practitioner – i.e. asking permission of the young person to inform parents or caregivers and what they are comfortable with.

Conclusion: Continuing the conversation

Conversations around mental health and wellbeing are becoming part of the mainstream, and broader conversation across society. The need to ensure Pacific people are part of these conversations is an important factor of also promoting wellbeing across our communities. This includes the meaningful inclusion of Pacific perspectives in the work we undertake as social workers across all fields of practice, but more so even more important to include when navigating the complexities associated with the impact across the family of an individual who is experiencing the effects of a mental illness. More work needs to be done across research and policy to assist governments and their systemic responses with ensuring good practice approaches are employed and utilised to enhance localised, regional and international approaches for Pacific people within the Oceania region and their diaspora globally.

> **REFLECTIVE QUESTIONS**
>
> 1. How would you differ your approach to working with Pacific families in the context of mental health and wellbeing?
> 2. What are some appropriate questions you could use to explore a family's understanding to assist in your ability to provide adequate resources to support their loved one with a mental illness?
> 3. How could you practically use concepts of *talanoa* and *Vā* as a means to develop meaningful conversations with Pacific individuals/families/groups about the prevalence and impact of mental illnesses? Could the use of *talanoa* and *Vā* also assist as a form of promoting effective recovery too?

References

Ataera-Minster, J. & Trowland, H. (2018). *Te Kaveinga: Mental health and wellbeing of Pacific peoples. Results from the New Zealand Mental Health Monitor & Health and Lifestyles Survey.* Retrieved from www.hpa.crg.nz

Connolly, M., Harms, L. & Maidment, J. (2018). *Social work: Contexts and practice* (4th Ed.). South Melbourne, Australia: Oxford University Press.

Han, H., Nicholas, A., Aimer, M. & Gray, J. (2015). An innovative community organizing campaign to improve mental health and wellbeing among Pacific Island youth in South Auckland, New Zealand. *Australasian Psychiatry: Bulletin of Royal Australian and New Zealand College of Psychiatrists*, 23(6), 670–674. https://doi.org/10.1177/1039856215597539

Le Va. (2017). *Kato Fetu: Review of the Pacific mental health and addiction research agenda.* Auckland. Retrieved from www.leva.co.nz/uploads/files/resources/Kato-Fetu-review-of-the-Pacific-mental-health-and-addiction-research-agenda.pdf

Mila-Schaaf, K. (2006). Vā-centred social work: Possibilities for a Pacific approach to social work practice. *Social Work Review*, 18(1), 8–13.

Mila-Schaaf, K. & Hudson, M. (2009). *Negotiating space for indigenous theorising in Pacific mental health and addictions.* Auckland, New Zealand. Retrieved from http://scholar.google.com/scholar?hl=en&btnG=Search&q=intitle:Negotiating+Space+for+Indigenous+Theorising+in+Pacific+Mental+Health+and+Addictions#0

Pacific Community. (2015). *Pacific Community Strategic Plan 2016–2020.* Noumea. Retrieved from www.spc.int/wp-content/uploads/2016/11/Strategic-Plan-2016-2020.pdf

Pacific Community. (2018). *SPC – Our work.* Retrieved from www.spc.int/about-us/our-work

Smith, M. & Jury, A. F. (2017). *Workforce development theory and practice in the mental health sector.* Hershey, PA: IGI Global.

Social Policy Evaluation and Research Unit. (2016). *Going digital to deliver wellbeing services to young people? Insights from e-tools supporting youth mental health and parenting.* Wellington, New Zealand. Retrieved from www.superu.govt.nz/publication/what_works_going_digital

Tonga National Health and Disabilities Association. (2017). *Langi Ma'a: Inaugural Tonga National Mental Health Symposium.* Retrieved from www.tmhdatonga.org/

Vaka, S., Brannelly, T., & Huntington, A. (2016). Getting to the heart of the story: Using Talanoa to explore Pacific mental health. *Issues in Mental Health Nursing, 37*(8), 537–544. https://doi.org/10.1080/01612840.2016.1186253

Vanuatu Ministry of Health. (2016). *Vanuatu mental health policy and strategic plan (2016–2020)*. Port Vila, Vanuatu: Vanuatu Ministry of Health.

Suggested further readings/websites

Ataera-Minster, J. & Trowland, H. (2018). *Te Kaveinga: Mental health and wellbeing of Pacific peoples. Results from the New Zealand Mental Health Monitor & Health and Lifestyles Survey*. Wellington, New Zealand: Health Promotion Agency. www.hpa.org.nz/sites/default/files/FinalReport-TeKaveinga-Mental%20health%20and%20wellbeing%20of%20Pacific%20peoples-Jun2018.pdf

Braam, A. W. (2017). Towards a multidisciplinary guideline religiousness, spirituality, and psychiatry: What do we need? *Mental Health, Religion and Culture, 20*(6), 579–588. https://doi.org/10.1080/13674676.2017.1377949

Charlson, F., Redman-MacLaren, M. & Hunter, E. (2015). Evaluation of a leadership in mental health course for Pacific Island Nation delegates. *Australasian Psychiatry, 23*(6), 38–41. https://doi.org/10.1177/1039856215612977

Faleafa, M. & Pulotu-Endemann, K. (2017). Developing a culturally competent workforce that meets the needs of Pacific people in New Zealand. In M. Smith and A. Jury (Eds.), *Workforce development theory and practice in the mental health sector* (pp. 165–180). IGI Global.

Headspace is a federally funded service in Australia that helps young people access mental health and wellbeing services through its community-based centres and online resources: https://headspace.org.au/

Kingi-'Uluave, D., Faleafa, M., Brown, T. & Daniela-Wong, E. (2007). Connecting culture and care: Clincial practice with Pasifika people. In I. Evans, J. Rucklidge, & M. O'Driscoll (Eds.), *Professional practice of psychology in Aotearoa New Zealand* (pp. 67–79). Wellington, New Zealand: New Zealand Psychological Society.

LeVa has a broad range of resources to, as per their mission, "support Pasifika families and communities to unleash their full potential and have the best possible health and wellbeing outcomes": www.leva.co.nz/

Mulder, R. T., Petaia, L., Pulotu-Endemann, F. K., Tuitama, G. L., Viali, S. & Parkin, I. (2015). Building on the strengths of Pacific mental health: Experience from Samoa. *Australian and New Zealand Journal of Psychiatry, 50*(5), 397–398. https://doi.org/10.1177/0004867415625816

Rodriguez, L. (2013). The subjective experience of Polynesians in the Australian health system. *Health Sociology Review, 22*(4), 411–421. https://doi.org/10.5172/hesr.2013.22.4.411

Vaka, S., Brannelly, T. & Huntington, A. (2016). Getting to the heart of the story: Using Talanoa to explore Pacific mental health. *Issues in Mental Health Nursing, 37*(8), 537–544. https://doi.org/10.1080/01612840.2016.1186253

6
ENVIRONMENTAL JUSTICE AND SOCIAL WORK IN CLIMATE CHANGE IN THE PACIFIC ISLANDS

Dora Kuir-Ayius and David Marena

Key points

- Climate change will continue to have an impact on the most vulnerable and marginalised communities in the Pacific.
- It is important to undertake a proactive stance on preparing people groups to risk manage consequences of climate change.
- Learning from indigenous approaches within environmental social work can benefit communities.
- This includes the need to uphold traditional cultural values whilst understanding the impact on losing access to traditional land and waters.

Introduction

Climate change is a major challenge in the 21st century as its impacts are great throughout the world. The effect of this issue varies in accordance mainly by its geographical location as different countries' weather patterns vary, as in the case of those in the Artic and Antarctica who experience a faster rate of melting ice while those in the tropics and low-lying islands face rising sea levels and other climate-related challenges. This chapter will explore the impact of climate change on Pacific Island Countries (PICs) through a social work lens by the application of theories in practical experiences in different island contexts. After this introduction, the chapter is divided into five sections comprised of understanding the international context of climate change, policy framework and application in the Pacific Islands, analysis of case studies, application of social work theories and climate change in the PICs and then a conclusion is given.

Understanding the international context of climate change

It is internationally agreed by the scientific community that climate change will pose one of the major challenges of this century (Mearns, 2010). People within different organisations including governments, international institutions and non-governmental organisations are concerned about these changes and, as such, have carried out studies to confirm the varying impacts of these changes in different parts of the world. A study on the impacts of climate change on world heritage sights on biodiversity of glaciers, marine, terrestrial, archaeological sites and historical cities (Colette, 2007) throughout the world revealed the threat posed by changes in climate. These studies in the different research locations clearly illustrated the impact of climate change melting glaciers, sea temperature changes and climate change forcing animal and plant species to migrate to other locations as they are unable to cope in their original environment (Colette, 2007). Each of its components is closely tied to adaptation objectives and aims to work in collaboration with stakeholders to assist impacted populations to effectively deal with climate change. Countries around the world have taken the issue of climate change as a challenge but see it as an opportunity to build and expound on existing partnerships, as in the case of the International Association of Schools of Social Work (IASSW) working in partnership with relevant stakeholders, including professionals from physical sciences, to deal with climate change and other issues (Dominelli, 2014a).

Policy framework and application in the Pacific Islands

In the Pacific Islands, there are several important strategic plans and other standards (see Table 6.1) that guide the management of climate change.

These standards are supported by the Information and Knowledge Management for Climate Change (IKM4CC) Strategic Framework developed in

TABLE 6.1 Climate change policy frameworks and programmes for PICs

Policies at regional level	National level
• Strategy for Climate and Disaster Resilient Development in the Pacific (Pacific Community, 2014). • Pacific Islands Framework for Action on Climate Change 2006–2015. • Disaster Risk Reduction and Management: A Framework for Action 2005–2015 (South Pacific Community, 2005). • Information and Knowledge Management for Climate Change (IKM4CC) Strategic Framework (Griffith University & Secretariat of the Pacific Regional Environment Program, 2016).	• 2007 National Climate Change Policy Framework (Fiji). • Tonga Strategic Development Framework (Tonga). • Strategic Program for Climate Change (PNG).

2016 by Griffith University and Secretariat of the Pacific Regional Environment Program (SPREP) in consultation with government representatives from Fiji, Vanuatu and Tonga who worked in the areas of climate change, disaster risk management and environmental management. This strategic framework provides a vision and pathway to assist in accessing well developed information management practices to deal with situations arising from climate change in PICs.

Social workers can facilitate between the different levels of governments and stakeholders and develop strategies to foster sustainable communities (Drolet & Sampson, 2017). This is evident in the way each of the PICs have developed policies to guide them to manage the impacts of climate change. Most of these policies are formulated in alignment with international frameworks including the previously prescribed United Nations' (UN's) Millennium Development Goals (MDGs) and the current Sustainable Development Goals (SDGs). Fiji, for example, in 2007 had its cabinet endorse its first ever National Climate Change Policy Framework that defined the "position of government and other stakeholders on issues of climate change, climate variability and sea level rise" (Government of the Republic of Fiji, 2012, p. v). This framework was reviewed in 2011 to address the current and emerging issues on climate change in alignment with its 2011 Corporate Plan of the Department of Environment providing a platform for partners to work on climate change mitigation and adaptation. This multi-sectoral approach is taken to emphasise UN's 1992 Agenda 21 which emphasised on inter-governmental cooperation.

The PICs have policy frameworks at both regional and national levels. The Pacific Islands Framework for Action on Climate Change 2006–2015 was observed when the different countries within the region planned and implemented programmes and projects including rising sea level as shown in the compendium (Secretariat of the Pacific Community et al., 2015). Other supporting frameworks such as the IKM4CC Strategic Framework are in place to play an assisting role in dealing with issues relating to climate change. Examples from case studies across the PICs emphasising on how people cope with the impacts of climate change in the environment are related to environmental social work as this is assisting "humanity to create and sustain a biodiverse ecosystem and does this by adapting existing social work methods" (Ramsay & Boddy, 2017. p. 68).

In the case of Papua New Guinea (PNG), the majority of its people rely heavily on the natural environment for their livelihood. Most Papua New Guineans depend on subsistence agriculture to support themselves. Therefore, the state joined the Coalition of Rainforest Nations (CfRN) in 2005. The PNG government has now gone ahead and formulated several policies through the Office of Climate Change and have formulated the National Climate Compatible Development Management Policy (GoPNG, 2014) in consultation with relevant stakeholders. This policy originated from the National Constitution, emphasising on the fourth goal, which focuses on natural resources and environment. This policy provides a clear pathway on the roles and responsibilities for coordination, implementation and review of climate change frameworks in the country. This policy's mission is to "build a climate resilient and carbon neutral pathway for climate compatible development in Papua New Guinea" (GoPNG, 2014, p. 8). This mission statement is the guide to programmes and projects concerning the impacts of climate change and implementation in PNG.

It is important to see if these strategies contributed to the building of resilience through cultural approaches to assist people to cope with the impact of climate change in the PICs.

Participatory cultural approaches to build resilient and sustainable communities

Participatory cultural approaches in building resilient and sustainable communities are important to the PICs. A compendium of Case Studies on Climate and Disaster Resilient Development in the Pacific (2015) profiled 40 case studies (Secretariat of the South Pacific Community, 2015) in the form of projects and programmes employed by different groups of people and organisations within the Pacific Islands to deal with the impacts of climate change. Two main themes from the case studies were: (1) the application of participatory and inclusive approaches to most vulnerable groups and (2) value of integrating gender perspectives in project development. Many of these case studies demonstrated participatory and inclusive approaches to those who were more vulnerable. A majority of these case studies also demonstrated the value of integrating gender aspects recognising the significance of "different roles, contributions, priorities and needs of women and men" (Secretariat of the South Pacific Community et al., 2015, p. 3). The compendium of the region also highlighted many other issues including geographical isolation, ecological fragility, lack of access and communication and setbacks caused by natural hazards (Secretariat of the South Pacific Community et al., 2015).

There is growing agreement that sustainable development in the PICs could be achieved through equal participation of men and women in project development. Projects on integrating gender equality through climate change must consider gender roles relating to traditional roles of men and women. A case study in Vanuatu on integrating gender equality in climate change programmes enabled men and women to work in partnership. Roles in a Melanesian country like Vanuatu are defined by gender, i.e. tasks that require more physical strength are generally done by men while women do other tasks to support such activities. For example, tasks involving the building of houses after natural disasters are executed mainly by men and women assist in preparing grass or palm leaves for roofing. There is a clear distinction between men and women in their roles and responsibilities. Therefore, it is vital to integrate indigenous gender perspectives in activities addressing climate change, in turn reiterating everyone's contribution within a collective context.

Climate change, vulnerability and relocation

Climate change creates vulnerable environments that lead to relocation. A study on vulnerability, adaptation and economic impact of climate change revealed several scenarios including rising sea levels, increase in surface air temperature, changes in rainfall, increase in the frequency of El Nino-related conditions and increase in the intensity of cyclones in the PICs (Chu, 2004). There are many competing definitions on the concept of vulnerability, but in this context we refer to lack of power, influence and control of those affected by climate change. This lack of power is reflected where access to resources are lessened because of rising sea levels, flooding rivers or landslide and other effects of climate change. In the PICs, including Kiribati, Vanuatu, Marshal Islands and Cook Islands, the chances of accessing basic needs such as food, water and land for survival are threatened.

Within the PICs, those affected by rising sea levels struggle to survive in severely damaged environments. Therefore, these people are forced to adapt to changes in their environment. Adaptation is a closely related concept to vulnerability in the context of disasters and survival of living organisms to survive in a physical environment in relation to each other's functions (Deutsch, Folke & Skånberg, 2003). The survival of an organism is influenced by the actions of other organisms that are competing for survival in the same environment. The successful survivors are the ones with a greater ability to adapt to disturbance while the vulnerable, with lesser capacity to withstand the pressures of change, typically vanish. More holistically, it is defined as a system "achieving desirable states in the face of change" (Engle, 2011, p. 649). It is likely that many systems encounter disturbances, but the important feature of resilient systems across human societies is that they can adapt or maintain their usual operations in the face of these disturbances.

Resilience, therefore, controls the extent to which a system can undergo changes before it encounters a disturbance that takes it to another stage where it can again stabilise around a new equilibrium. This is closely related to the concept of adaptability, which can be defined as the learning aspect of a system that copes with the disturbances that have occurred (Deutsch et al., 2003). The more this system can adapt the more resilient it is. Therefore, the concepts of adaptability and resilience are intimately related. The resilience of people affected by the rising sea levels and other climate change effects must be taken into consideration to address the issues in a most relevant manner, including policy formulations and programme implementation.

Transformation of the land by rising sea levels in fact changes the environment to a different system (Walker et al., 2009) where you have less land available for human habitation. Transformations in ecology typically refer to processes that occur in response to harm or repeated negative experiences of the system (McDonald, 2007). Such systems including land drowned by the rising sea levels have undergone continuous negative encounters that have destroyed their original state. These aspects of resilience become significant when there is continuous negativity or undesirable processes impacting on the stability of a system, adaptability is no longer possible within the system to survive and therefore it needs transformation (Folke, 2006).

Some governments of PICs have considered relocation as an alternative to save populations affected by rising sea levels and other impacts of climate change. However, relocation of people from a PIC's perspective does have negative implications on all stakeholders including the immigrants, landowners of resettlement area and the government. Land is communally owned and valuable to the survival of people.

Generally, land in the PICs is communally owned by clans or tribes; its use is highly valued. Rising sea levels take over land previously used for gardening and villages, forcing these people to seek refuge elsewhere. For example, within the PICs, including Kiribati, Papua New Guinea and Fiji, many homes that were situated along the sea shore are now under water. In PNG, the Carteret and Mortlock Islands are sinking through rising sea levels. The plight of Carteret islanders to resettle on Bougainville has been persistent but only achieved through the assistance of the Catholic Diocese of Bougainville who provided land. This outcome is the result of continuous efforts of Tulele Peisa, a local non-government organization (NGO) who negotiated for resettlement of the islanders.

The issue of landownership is one of the most complicated in Melanesia as illustrated in the mining context and has contributed to numerous conflicts (Kuir-Ayius, 2016). This as Jorgensen (1997) argues is due to three main reasons: numerous claimants to pieces of land, complex land histories giving rise to claims from conflicting clans and the state's recognition of indigenous land rights giving rise to pressure by these landowners in the state.

Land ownership in PNG is also complicated by people's oral histories and social identities, and their connections to the physical land features. Land is a "shorthand for ties to locality – whether terrestrial or marine – [and] is the basis for membership and nationality for most Melanesians" (Ballard, 2013, p. 48). Examples of landownership in mine-affected communities are no different from other non-mining communities. Resources are deeply connected to the creation and continuation of kinship relations and identity of people (Banks, 2008). This can cause complications in separating people from the physical features they associate their identity with, and in turn this can affect the delivery of infrastructure and services when landownership is contested. Relocation of populations impacted by climate change will pose risks of creating land issues in PICs.

Jorgensen's (1997) argument that the state's recognition of indigenous land rights gives rise to different claims regarding the benefits of mining is true in the sense that the indigenous people argue for their rights to the benefits of mining. There have been cases where landowners demand compensation and put the developer under pressure to meet these demands outside the scope of the Memorandum of Agreement for the operation. This view is supported by Filer (1990), who describes the ultimatums of landowners in Bougainville who demanded an enormous 10-billion-kina compensation from the company for environmental damages; when this was not forthcoming, violence followed and the mine closed. Dove et al. (as cited by Banks, 2008, p. 25) summarise the significance of land and therefore highlight the importance of landownership, "[l]and is our life. And our physical life-food and sustenance. Land is our social life; it is marriage; it is status; it is security; it is policies; in fact it is our only world".

Indigenous landowner issues are complicated as people's livelihoods are associated to their environment. In many cases in Melanesia, the signing of a Memorandum of Agreement (MoA) does not always stop people from demanding additional revenues and benefits. Land rights issues in PNG and other PICs cannot be eliminated but they can be managed to a level where benefits are shared more equally among all parties.

Environmental social work and climate change in the PICs

Environmental social work has a part to play in protecting the non-human (Gray & Coates, 2012). The concept is "founded on ecological justice principles" (Ramsay & Boddy, 2017, p. 68). An ecological understanding on environmental social work requires a partnership approach from all stakeholders. In environmental justice, environmental social work widens the understanding on the impact of climate change on the poorest and marginalised populations. For instance, it is important for social workers to directly work with traditional landowners, empowering them to make informed decisions as to what to do if they are relocated. Poverty continues to be one of the major drivers of environmental destruction as the poor lack choices in developed cities while the very poor in the South depend heavily on the environment for survival (Gray & Coates, 2012). This is clearly evident in the PICs as most people depend heavily on the land and the sea for food.

Climate change through rising sea levels also threaten loss of certain cultural values. There is fear of losing cultural values through emigrations from village elders of the Mortlock Islands within PNG. The Carteret islanders face difficulties in replicating their island environment to their relocated land on the main island of Bougainville. These islanders are among the few PICs who have been relocated. Tulele Peisa continues to work in partnership with others to preserve and protect the culture and biodiversity of the Carteret islanders. Given the challenges posed by climate change, there seem to be lack of evidence on social work research in this subject (Kemp, 2011). Due to their geographical isolation, they sustain their livelihood through the sea and its resources. However, climate change through rising sea levels diminishes these islanders' resilience, causing these people to be dependent on external assistance from the government and other partners outside of their island. Such low-lying land seen across the Carteret and Mortlock Islands in PNG and people in Lau Lagoon on Malaita, Solomon Islands are illustrations of growing dependence among the impacted populations on outsiders for survival.

Climate change is an environmental crisis that exacerbates political, socio-economic and cultural inequalities (Dominelli, 2014a). Disasters in the form of flooding and hurricane-type strong winds contribute to the destruction of property and crops that are important to a community's livelihood. The PICs are vulnerable to this type of environmental crisis since they are among the most affected groups of people in the world.

Therefore, social workers can positively assist PICs who are impacted by climate change. As such, environmental social work has a role in challenging governments, non-governmental organisations, civil society and international organisations to protect the environment. Social work and social development can be places to work effectively in collaboration with stakeholders globally. There is a need for social workers – both practitioners and educators – to develop new skills to strategise, advocate and invest in people and the PICs and build organisational and community capacity, including challenges caused by climate change, to create resilient and sustainable communities (Pacific Islands Forum Fisheries Agency [FFA], 2018). Social workers in and across the Pacific region, especially educators, lack research and publications on climate change in the PICs and would benefit from having such knowledge to further support the practical applications of strategies and other forms of assistance needed to counteract the seriousness and real challenges being experienced.

Conclusion

Climate change is a global phenomenon that is negatively impacting communities around the world, and the PICs are no exception. The different PICs have developed policies that align with global standards to deal with challenges brought upon them. Analysis of case studies illustrated that these island nations have different programmes to prepare affected populations in dealing with climate change. This chapter has viewed programmes within the PICs in the perspective of environmental social work and its application of chosen theories in various PICs in the context of climate change. Discussions also focused on the significance of equal participation of men and women through the resilience of cultural approaches that contributes to the building of sustainable communities. Social work plays a significant role in empowering those who are disadvantaged by climate change. Social workers, both educators and practitioners, must participate in assisting those negatively affected by climate change in the Pacific region.

References

Arnold, M., Mearns, R., Oshima, K. & Prasad, V. (2016). Climate and disaster resilience. *World Bank*, 70.

Ballard, C. (2013). It's the land, stupid! The moral economy of resource ownership in Papua New Guinea. In P. Larmour (Ed.), *The governance of common property in the Pacific region* (pp. 47–65).

Banks, G. (2008). Understanding "resource" conflicts in Papua New Guinea. *Asia Pacific Viewpoint 49*(1), 23–34.

Deutsch, L., Folke, C. & Skånberg, K. (2003). The critical natural capital of ecosystem performance as insurance for human well-being. *Ecological Economics*, *44*(2–3), 205–217.

Dominelli, L. (2014a). Promoting environmental justice through green social work practice: A key challenge for practitioners and educators. *International Social Work*, *57*(4), 338–345.

Dominelli, L. (2014b). Learning from our past: Climate change and disaster interventions in practice. In C. Noble, H. Strauss and B. Littlechild (Eds.), *Global social work* (pp. 341–351). Sydney, Australia: Sydney University Press.

Drolet, J. L. & Sampson, T. (2017). Addressing climate change from a social development approach: Small cities and rural communities' adaptation and response to climate change in British Columbia, Canada. *International Social Work*, *60*(1), 61–73.

Engle, N. L. (2011). Adaptive capacity and its assessment. *Global Environmental Change*, *21*(2), 647–656.

Filer, C. (1990). The Bougainville rebellion, the mining industry and the process of social disintegration in Papua New Guinea. *Canberra Anthropology*, *13*(1), 1–39.

Folke, C. (2006). Resilience: The emergence of a perspective for social–ecological systems analyses. *Global Environmental Change*, *16*(3), 253–267.

GoPNG. (2014). *National climate compatible development management policy*. Port Moresby, Papua New Guinea: Author.

Government of the Republic of Fiji. (2012). *Republic of Fiji national climate change policy*. Suva, Fiji: Secreteriat of the Pacific Community.

Gray, M. & Coates, J. (2012). Environmental ethics for social work: Social work responsibility to the non-human world. *International Journal of Social Welfare*, *21*(3), 239–247.

Griffith University & Secretariat of the South Pacific Regional Environment Program. (2016). *Information and knowledge management for climate change (IKM4CC) guidelines: Complete set*. Brisbane, Australia: Authors.

Jorgensen, D. (1997). Who and what is a landowner? Mythology and marking the ground in a Papua New Guinea mining project. *Anthropological Forum*, *7*(4), 599–627.

Kemp, S. P. (2011). Recentring environment in social work practice: Necessity, opportunity, challenge. *British Journal of Social Work*, *41*(6), 1198–1210.

Kuir-Ayius, D. (2016). *Building community resilience in mine-impacted communities: A study on delivery of health services in Papua New Guinea* (unpublished doctoral dissertation). Massey University, Palmerston North, New Zealand.

McDonald, T. (2007). Resilience thinking: Interview with Brian Walker. *Journal of Ecological Management and Restoration*, *8*(2), 85–91.

Mearns, L. O. (2010). Quantification of uncertainties of future climate change: Challenges and applications. *The Philosophy of Science Association*, *77*(55), 131–143.

Pacific Islands Forum Fisheries Agency (FFA). (2018). *Regional Organisations in the Pacific*. Retrieved from www.ffa.int/regional_organisations

Ramsay, S. & Boddy, J. (2017). Environmental social work: A concept analysis. *British Journal of Social Work*, *47*, 68–86.

Secretariat of the Pacific Regional Programme (2005). Pacific Islands framework for action on climate change 2006–2015. (2nd ed.). Apia, Samoa: Author.

Secretariat of the South Pacific Community et al. (2015). *Compendium of case studies on climate and disaster resilient development in the Pacific*. Suva, Fiji: Author.

South Pacific Community. (2005). *Disaster risk reduction and disaster management: a framework for action 2005–2015: An investment for sustainable development in the Pacific Island Countries*. Suva, Fiji: Author

Walker, B. H., Abel, N., Anderies, J. M. & Ryan, P. (2009). Resilience, adaptability, and transformability in the Goulburn-Broken Catchment, Australia. *Ecology & Society*, *14*(1), 12.

Suggested further readings/websites

Climate Change and Food Security in Pacific Island Countries: www.fao.org/climate change/17003-02529d2a5afee62cce0e70d2d38e1e273.pdf

Climate Change Scenarios in the Pacific: http://siteresources.worldbank.org/INTP ACIFICISLANDS/Resources/4-Chapter+2.pdf

Compendium of Case Studies on Climate Change and Disaster Resilient Development in the Pacific: https://reliefweb.int/report/world/compendium-case-studies-climate-and-disaster-resilient-development-pacific-2015

National Climate Compatible Development Management policy: http://d3605781.u199.pngconnect.com/images/National%20Climate%20Compatible%20Development%20Management.pdf

Republic of Kiribati Island Report Series: climate.gov.ki

The Global Agenda for Social Work and Social Development: www.globalsocial agenda.org

7

PACIFIC-INDIGENOUS COMMUNITY-VILLAGE RESILIENCE IN DISASTERS

Siautu Alefaio-Tugia, Emeline Afeaki-Mafile'o and Petra Satele

Key points

- Whilst Pacific nations experience natural disasters exacerbated by climate change, Pacific enactment of family-reliance including the transnational Pacific diaspora demonstrates Pacific-Indigenous community-village resilience.
- Pacific-Indigenous communities traditionally possessed knowledges and practices (related to food security, built environment and social structures) which enabled preparation, recovery and adaptation to disasters.
- Responses to the Samoa tsunami in 2009 demonstrate *fa'asinomaga*, an others-centredness, and culturally-informed responses.
- Responses to Cylone Gita in Tonga in 2018 demonstrate the role of social entrepreneurship and partnerships in recovery and preparedness.

Introduction

The Pacific is one of the most natural disaster-prone regions on earth ('Aho, 2018). Pacific Island countries are vulnerable to natural hazards that include floods, droughts, tropical cyclones, earthquakes, volcanic eruptions and tsunamis. In the disaster context, resilience and vulnerability go hand in hand. When a shock or disturbance arises, such as a disaster, a resilient individual or group are able to purposefully identify, access and utilise available resources. Throughout the field of climate change, disaster risk resilience and disaster risk management, resilience is a commonly used term yet defined in several different ways. Definitions of resilience include the ability and capacity for an individual or group to adapt and respond to risk. In other words, "to navigate their way to the psychological, social, cultural, and physical resources that sustain their wellbeing, and their capacity individually and collectively to negotiate for these resources to be provided and experienced in culturally meaningful ways" (Paton and Johnston, 2017, p. 139). Disaster resilience has been interpreted as a process of recovery and self-learning (Aldunce et al., 2015, p. 2). It is the importance of being able to "return to baseline functioning" after a disaster (Aldunce et al., 2015, p. 2). It is not only about returning to the state before the disturbance, but advancing through "learning and adaptation" (Cutter et al., 2008, p. 3). Some definitions of resilience focus on the preparation aspect, rather than just recovery. It is important to have a "capacity to anticipate, prepare and plan in order to recover from the negative impacts of a hazard and to mitigate, prevent and minimize losses, suffering and social disruption" (Aldunce et al., 2015, p. 2). Closely tied to this idea is self-reliance, which is an important part of being resilient. Self-reliance is being able to survive, while not being overly dependent on help from others. This chapter recognises the ambiguity of the term resilience (Alexander, 2013) in the field of disaster risk resilience, management and climate change, and provides a Pacific-Indigenous perspective to the context through two case studies, one based in Samoa and the other in Tonga. For example, the idea of "self-reliance" as the ability to survive while not being overly dependent on others relates to the notion of "kinship". As highlighted by the former Head of State of Samoa Tupua Tamasese Efi (2009) during his address post-tsunami, "*O lē e lave i tigā, ole ivi, le toto, ma le aano*" (He who rallies in my hour of need is my kin). Dependency for survival during crises for those born in the Islands – Samoa and the Kingdom of Tonga – is upon their own "kin" (family). Within the Pacific-Indigenous context, *family-reliance* as opposed to "self-reliance" is enacted. Families across the globe in new worlds of Pacific-diasporic settlement provide familial-reliance and resiliency to sustain families back home in their Island nations.

The case studies in this chapter illustrate the catastrophic effects on our vulnerable islands; Samoa in 2009 when devastated by a tsunami on its South-West coast and most recently Cyclone Gita that hit the Kingdom of Tonga in 2018. These examples illustrate how globalisation has compounded the effects of climate change and is likely to increase the vulnerability of our Pacific nations. In the midst of this vulnerability, resilience is prevalent through *family-reliance* on Pacific diaspora who ensure the return of families in their Island-home nations to "everyday" functioning. The impact of families mobilising through the Pacific diaspora demonstrates Pacific-Indigenous community-village resilience.

CASE STUDY 7.1: SAMOA

Galuega toe Fuata'ina – Samoa tsunami 2009

Galuega toe Fuata'ina, a Samoan metaphorical proverb, was used by the Cultural-Elder Advisors of SUNGO (Samoa Umbrella of Non-Governmental Organisations) to describe and capture the psycho-social response work undertaken by many local and overseas volunteers, support workers and professionals brought together by the sudden *Mala Fa'anatura* (natural disaster) that struck Samoa on September 29, 2009. The essence of *Galuega toe Fuata'ina* is perhaps best described through the Samoan poetical proverbial expression *Toe timata le upega*. The expression metaphorically relates a fishing analogy, to *rethinking* and *reflecting* on crisis in *motion*, to try again, to do it again in order to start again. It has a restorative destination in mind. The process, however, is naturally painful. The collective village resilience that was called on during Samoa's tsunami is captured poignantly by Samoa's former Head of State Tui Atua Tupua Tamasese Ta'isi Efi. He described the tsunami of September 29 as being *"potent not only for the death and destruction it caused, but also, as has been the case throughout history, for the invitation to reassess, cleanse and make anew"*. This is akin to adaptation within the societal system using resources to learn, change, reorganise and be innovative (Adger et al., 2011, p. 757; Cutter et al., 2008, p. 3).

Fa'asinomaga is a central tenet of Samoan cultural identity and is conceptualised as one's inheritance designated by the designator – God. This designation is located in the heart, mind and soul of a person. It is what gives one meaning and belonging. It is what defines ways of relating to others (*vā fealoaloa'i*) and boundaries (*tua'oi*) between one's self and others, one and the environment, one and the cosmos and a person and God (Alefaio-Tugia, 2015). An infamous metaphorical depiction of *fa'asinomaga* is captured poignantly by one of Samoa's foremost cultural guardians – Tui Atua Tupua Tamasese Ta'isi Efi:

> I am not an individual; I am an integral part of the cosmos. I share divinity with my ancestors, the land, the seas and the skies. I am not an individual, because I share a tofi (inheritance) with my family, my village and my nation. I belong to my family and my family belongs to me. I belong to my village and my village belongs to me. I belong to my nation and my nation belongs to me. This is the essence of my sense of belonging.
>
> *(Efi, 2003)*

Disaster response in a society such as Samoa whose *fa'asinomaga* (essence of life) is centred in "others" or "*others-centered*" (Alefaio-Tugia, 2015) takes on a form that is organically collectively-resilient. Therefore, the general understanding within the context of natural disasters of community resilience being the ability to overcome extreme events without significant outside assistance (Cutter et al., 2008, p. 5) demonstrates how literature does not take into account Pacific-Indigenous ways of "knowing, being and doing" where shared *tofi* (inheritance) and *fa'asinomaga* (essence of life) calls on all Samoans no matter what geographical location they are living in to *respond to their kin*. Pacific-Indigenous cultural ways of "knowing, being and doing" collide with protocols of disaster response, recovery and management but often are key bridging elements for disaster risk resilience and sustainable recovery. During the immediate response to the Samoan tsunami, New Zealand sent teams filled with Samoan nurses, doctors and appropriate practitioners. The call went out for "Samoan-speaking" psychologists, of which I (Siautu) was one. The Pacific-Indigenous diaspora based in Aotearoa New Zealand identified the need for Samoan-speaking professionals. This highlights the organic and natural cultural-responsiveness enacted by Pacific-Indigenous diaspora. Having been born in New Zealand but raised by Samoan parents to speak Samoan and enact *Fa'aSamoa* (Samoan indigenous cultural protocols) during my "everyday", being back in Samoa was my "return home" (despite having been back physically many times before). The nation-hood distress call was heeded by many Samoans – whether they could speak Samoan or not, all responded. The impact on the field of disaster was immediate. I recall a fellow psychologist colleague that came from Australia commenting that she had never experienced being involved in a disaster where there was such an enormous amount of "cultural responsiveness" from professionals of the diasporic population, and especially those who spoke the language. As children of Samoa (whether born in Samoa or not, made little difference), *all* Samoans during the disaster heeded the *call* and responded collectively to the immediate needs. The advantage came in the ability as Samoans to understand local cultural protocols and thereby respond appropriately to the immediate needs.

Culturally responsive field innovations

As a Samoan-speaking psychologist practitioner engaged directly in immediate psycho-social response, I recognised that while there was a lack of "professionals" such as psychologists, psychiatrists and trauma counsellors, there were a plethora of locally appropriate and culturally relevant field-leaders such as church ministers/pastors and their wives, theological students and village Elders from unaffected parts of the nation who were already "on the ground" during the immediate response and were effectively utilising Samoan cultural protocols to bring immediate healing to families, villages and communities. Recognising and being aware that localised Samoan-indigenous responses were already in immediate-motion enabled the identification of those most appropriate to provide psychological first-aid and post-disaster follow-up. There would never be enough psychologists, trauma counsellors or social-workers as these professions do not exist in sufficient numbers in Samoa or throughout the Island nations. However, what exists within the social-cultural fabric of *Fa'aSamoa* (Samoan-Indigenous cultural knowledge) are the locally designated frontline crisis-workers: ministers, pastors, ministers'/pastors' wives, theological students. Identifying these as immediate first responders enabled training to occur across the various religious affiliations. All were welcomed to the training and provided follow-up resourcing to enable effective psycho-social response and recovery.

Samoa's former Head of State, Tui Atua Tupua's, address following the tsunami emphasised two sides of disaster – *potency* for the death and destruction and *opportunity* (or invitation) to *reassess, cleanse and make anew*. In the provision of psycho-social support through psychological first-aid, *cleansing* of "western" ideological forms of immediate response such as needing to call on more psychologists, trauma counsellors and social workers were alleviated through identifying those culturally relevant and appropriate, thereby creating *a new* body of first responders equipped locally. In Figure 7.1, a visual depiction of Pacific-Indigenous disaster response is illustrated. *Tama Fanau* (Children of the Pacific diaspora) are *carriers of indigenous knowledge* through the languages spoken and unspoken carried within their hearts. During critical times of disasters they are *facilitators of "communication-exchange"*. In one of the many debriefs with the medical teams, a concern was raised by medical officers around the burning of plastic water bottles provided by humanitarian aid agencies as the toxicity of the air was causing breathing difficulties for children and Elders. A nurse born in Samoa but living in New Zealand suggested

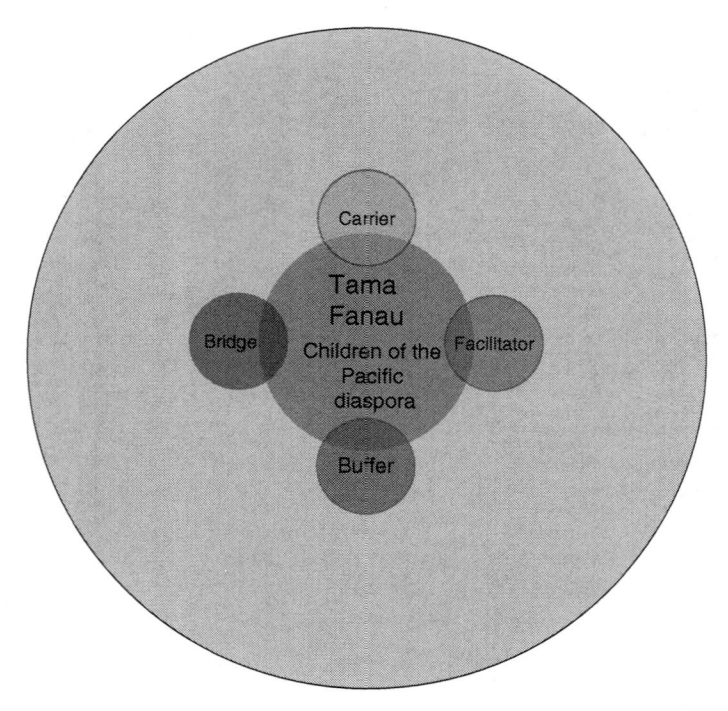

FIGURE 7.1 Pacific-Indigenous disaster response.

to put a call out to villages unaffected by the tsunami to "*koli mai niu*", gather as many niu (baby coconuts) known for their high nutritional properties and to use this as opposed to the water bottles. This is an example of culturally relevant communication-exchange during critical times. *Tama Fanau* are crucial in *bridging the cultural communication gap* that easily occurs during high intensity situations such as disasters where high-level decisions are made every day. They also *buffer cultural inappropriateness* from people and agencies that have descended as part of the humanitarian response.

Community resilience

Disaster resilience focusing on larger groups such as communities indicate that resilient groups or communities should theoretically be stronger after a disaster and more prepared to face another. In using traditional knowledge, key elements were focused on achieving sustainability and building resilience against disaster. Two of these elements were food security and settlement security (Campbell, 2009, p. 85). Food security was a key element in traditional disaster management. This was achieved through producing a surplus of food to be preserved and stored. Crops such as yams, taro and breadfruit could be stored underground in pits and left to ferment. This ensured that there was immediate food following a disaster, and whether it be a cyclone or tsunami, the food would be unaffected underground. Such strategies ensured that communities were prepared for potential disasters to wipe out some, or all, of their crops and they would be able to recover from the damage and thrive. Settlement security was another key element of traditional risk reduction, which included purposefully selecting areas to build up settlements, which were not close to coastlines, and were elevated. Early Europeans noted that the houses seemed disorganised, "an eyesore from the European perspective. But neat rows provide useful corridors for hurricane force winds to blow through and wreak havoc" (Campbell, 2009, p. 91). Houses were also built to be wind-resistant with few windows and doors, and sennit used to bind the structures together, instead of nails, allowing more flexibility and strength (Campbell, 2009). Unfortunately, through colonialism, development and globalisation many of these Pacific-Indigenous traditional practices have declined and become nonexistent, thereby increasing the vulnerability of Pacific-Indigenous communities to the wrath of natural weather extremes.

It is very important to note that throughout the Pacific, people were traditionally very resilient and had disaster risk reduction and management strategies in place. However, with the introduction of colonisation and cash economies, traditional knowledge economies have been displaced and created vulnerabilities within the social fabric of many Pacific nations. Social changes that came with colonialism and modernisation have affected these traditional practices. For example, food storage was affected when rice and cabin biscuits, among other imported food, was introduced (Campbell, 2009, p. 92). Today, many Pacific Island nations throughout Oceania rely heavily on government relief and aid when hit with disaster. However, Pacific-Indigenous ways of responding during and post-disaster involving the Pacific diaspora provide innovative ways for adapting to change. Families of Pacific peoples affected by disasters respond more immediately and with vigour than aid agencies and government support. The focus of this next case study showcases effective community-village resilience.

CASE STUDY 7.2: KINGDOM OF TONGA

It was not an accident that social worker, Emeline, the founder of Affirming Works (AW), a social service based in Auckland, New Zealand, was residing in Kolonga, Tongatapu when Cyclone Gita swept through the Kingdom of Tonga. Emeline and her husband set up businesses in Tonga and utilised entrepreneurial opportunities to provide social work services to Pacific communities. Community Café was set up in 2010 in Auckland, New Zealand, as a social enterprise with the purpose of breaking down silos between services in the community, providing a citizen-centric access point for all multi-cultural communities. Improved accessibility to existing services and encouraging a collaborative and co-operative response to community needs is the heart-beat of Community Café. In the same year, a coffee business in the Kingdom of Tonga was purchased, enabling an enterprising opportunity for the Tongan diaspora to work together to provide ways forward by building community-village resilience but also a more sustainable approach to development. With a social work background, I value promoting social change and development, social cohesion and the empowerment and liberation of people. Therefore, using Tongan-grown products manufactured in the homeland for the Pacific diaspora markets, specifically Aotearoa-New Zealand, we have created a new Pacific-Indigenous model of development that empowers locally owned and sustainable solutions for the liberation of our Pacific communities both in our Island-nations and the global diaspora.

Tupu'anga Coffee, named after Affirming Works (AW) flagship mentoring programme, provided the connection to the diaspora enabling new levels of resiliency. Through a partnership with Joint Centre for Disaster Research (JCDR), School of Psychology, Massey University, Tupu'anga Coffee hosted a strategic gathering in Tonga focused on disaster preparedness amongst the diaspora. The 2016 strategic gathering we hosted in Tonga developed organically with JCDR Director Professor David Johnston and students and staff including Dr Siautu Alefaio together with a delegate from Auckland Council, which represents the City with the largest Pacific population in the world. As a result of these initiatives, NIUPacH (New Indigenous Unity of Pacific Humanitarians), a virtual research collective, was formed by Dr Siautu Alefaio, who also created Talanoa HUBBS to help strengthen and mobilise existing Pacific-Indigenous diaspora – in our case, the Tongan-diaspora. Figure 7.2 illustrates the vision of Talnoa HUBBS hosted by Tupu'anga Café in Tonga. Figure 7.3 showcases participants in full-talanoa mode.

The impact of Pacific-Indigenous leadership and effective partnerships illustrates how we as Pacific diaspora have collectively taken responsibility for ensuring our communities build back better and stronger post-disaster. Social work literature highlights that "disaster is a trauma that occurs to a whole community" and is similar to the "collective traumatisation of indigenous people", therefore healing and intervention must be focused on the collective (Gray et al., cited in Pyles, 2017).

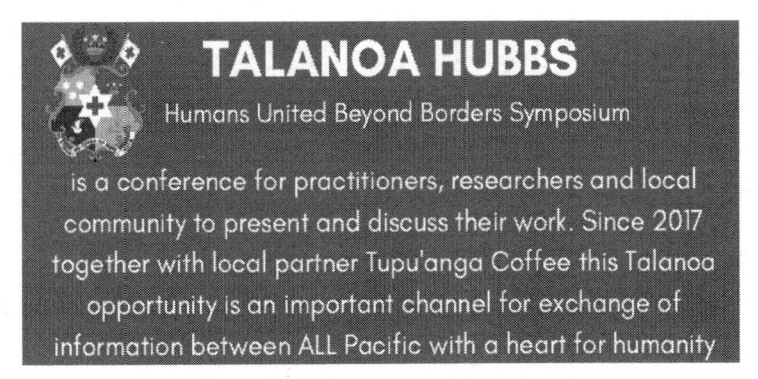

TALANOA HUBBS
Humans United Beyond Borders Symposium

is a conference for practitioners, researchers and local community to present and discuss their work. Since 2017 together with local partner Tupu'anga Coffee this Talanoa opportunity is an important channel for exchange of information between ALL Pacific with a heart for humanity

FIGURE 7.2   Vision of Talanoa HUBBS hosted in Tonga by Tupu'anga Café (Author).

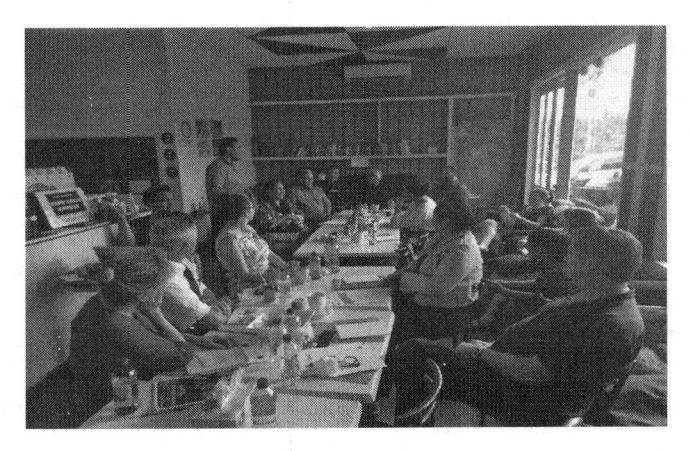

FIGURE 7.3   2017 Delegates in full talanoa-mode (Author).

We have continued to host gatherings in the Kingdom of Tonga at our Tupu'anga Café, growing annually in momentum and responsibility to ensure work in the Pacific develops more closely together. Despite being small Island-nations, fragmentation in our communities has resulted due to current development models and aid programmes. Every year the Tupu'anga Coffee factory hosts dignitaries from government, private sector, education, church and social services to ensure that communication and accessibility to good information is available to all. The *talanoa* dialogue with business owners, educators and government officials, which began as an organic response, was strategically effective as it emphasised the importance of a trans-disciplinary approach to developing a nation. This is important as disaster preparedness has to coincide with development of the nation.

In 2018, Cyclone Gita struck the Kingdom of Tonga on February 12, 2018. The areas most affected were Tongatapu and Eu'a; 75% (an estimated 80,000 people) were impacted with 800 households destroyed and 4,000 damaged. Despite essential services and public buildings affected there was no loss of life in the nation. The response from the diaspora was immediate, for example, there were calls on the radio for ex-employees of the Tongan power company to return to their homeland to assist in the repair of electricity poles. Their own family homes without power or even roofs were responded to by their extended family members abroad. Affirming Works became a conduit for Pacific-diaspora communities in Melbourne, Australia and Auckland, New Zealand to contribute to the Cyclone Gita disaster response in Tonga. Fundraising collaborations with an enterprising former student of the Tupu'anga mentoring programme living in Melbourne was hosted in the Community Café in New Zealand. We developed the #TagTonga initiative from these fundraising events with the aim to provide funds tagged by Pacific-diaspora directly to those (families, causes, projects) they selected. When Pacific-Indigenous diaspora mobilise and respond organically, it counteracts "disaster capitalism" phenomenon – profiteering and privatisation of social programmes during disasters (Pyles, 2017). If profiteering by Pacific-diaspora occurs, the weight of disappointment is felt by the collective-village communities and natural cultural justice is enacted. Spaces that provided a sense of connectedness and normality in Nuku'alofa such as cafés and restaurants became a place of comfort. This was the case for our Tupu'anga café/factory when community and church leaders and other private business owners would meet and share their experiences of preparing and responding to the disaster. The lack of food supplies meant heavy reliance on the overseas provision, and demand drove the cost of staple foods much higher. However, our orders for coffee and chips were bustling out the door despite the fact that most of Tonga, including ourselves (at home), were without power. My own reflection being present during the Cyclone was that it felt like a huge tourist event with the amount of people coming and going in Tonga. Oxfam emphasised the unintended consequences that occur during disasters when disaster relief and recovery are in full effect. Food, water and housing needs for relief workers as well as external foods and products flooding the local markets can all create a negative impact to the local economy. In our experience, during Cyclone Gita, the Tupu'anga Café/factory provided a place for refreshment (coffee and food), *talanoa* (organic and robust dialogue) and generations of new collaborations during disaster response and recovery.

Joining together to find ways to support each other during a critical time of need, as children were not in school and workplaces had not returned to normal rhythms, was our own Tongan-indigenous ways of resilience. The National Day of Prayer where the King of Tonga (King 'Aho'eitu Tupou VI) knelt and prayed was a significant act for a whole nation's cultural-faith resilience. The people of Tonga believe that God spared the nation from a category five cyclone. During the Talanoa HUBBS (see Figure 7.4) we hosted in May 2018, all these parties that frequented the café were invited to debrief their experiences and provide an indigenous experience to the current research on disasters in the Pacific. Presentations by Tonga's National Emergency Office (NEMO) and Met Service reinforced participant's beliefs that God spared Tonga as a nation from catastrophic destruction.

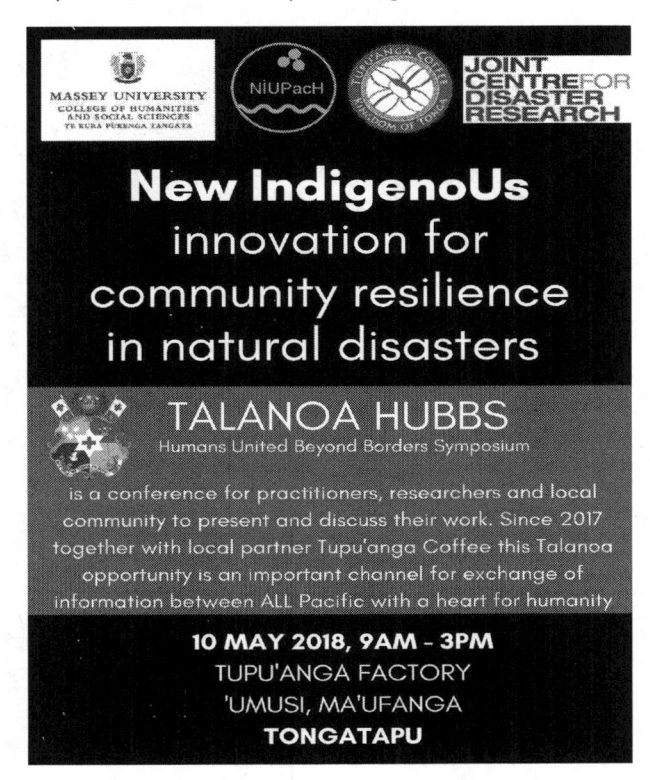

FIGURE 7.4   2018 Talanoa HUBBS in Tonga hosted by Tupu'anga Café (Author).

Conclusion

Overall, this chapter has provided a transnational focus to disaster response from a Pacific-Indigenous lens. The case studies have illustrated Pacific-Indigenous collective mobilisation during disasters and the impact children of the Pacific diaspora have as key drivers for mobilising effective response during disasters. In essence, Pacific-Indigenous community-village resilience in disasters underscores the importance for social work to be community-centred (Pyles, 2017) and contributes new knowledge in the context of disasters, humanitarian response and climate change.

References

Adger, W. N., Brown, K., Nelson, D. R., Berkes, F., Eakin, H., Folke, C., ... Tompkins, E. L. (2011). Resilience implications of policy responses to climate change. *Climate Change*, 2(5), 757–766.

'Aho, L. (2018). Tongan Cyclone Gita Response [PowerPoint slides]. National Emergency Management Office (NEMO). Talanoa HUBBS Tonga, 10 May 2018.

Aldunce, P., Beilin, R., Howden, M. & Handmer, J. (2015). Resilience for disaster risk management in a changing climate: Practitioners' frames and practices. *Global Environmental Change*, 30, 1–11.

Alefaio-Tugia, S. T. (2015). Galuola: A NIU way for informing psychology from the cultural context of Fa'aSamoa (Version 1). fighsare. https://doi.org/10.4225/03/58abad465cdc1

Alexander, D. E. (2013). Resilience and disaster risk reduction: An etymological journey. *Natural Hazards and Earth System Sciences*, 13, 2707–2716.

Campbell, J. (2009). Islandness: Vulnerability and resilience in Oceania. *Shima: The International Journal of Research into Island Cultures*, 3, 85–97.

Cutter, S. L., Barnes, L., Berry, M., Burton, C., Evans, E., Tate, E. & Webb, J. (2008). A place-based model for understanding community resilience to natural disasters. *Global Environmental Change*, 18(4), 598–606.

Efi, T. A. T. T. (2003). In search of meaning, nuance, and metaphor in social policy. *Social Policy Journal of New Zealand*, 20, 49–63.

Efi, T. A. T. T. (2009). Head of State of the Independent State of Samoa Keynote Address, New Zealand Families Commission Pasifika Families' Fono 3 November 2009, www.head-of-statesamoa.ws/speeches_pdf/Tupua%20Family%20Commission%20FINAL4%20(2).pdf

Paton, D. & Johnston, D. (2017). *Disaster resilience: An integrated approach*. Springfield, IL: Charles C Thomas Publisher LTD.

Pyles, L. (2017). Decolonising disaster social work: Environmental justice and community participation. *British Journal of Social Work*, 47(3), 630–647. doi:10.1093/bjsw/bcw028

8

DELIVERING YOUTH JUSTICE FOR PACIFIC YOUNG PEOPLE AND THEIR FAMILIES

Jioji Ravulo, Jack Scanlan and Vivian Koster

Key points

- Understanding the broader legal system and how it interacts with Pacific young people and their families is important in finding positive and practical solutions.
- Specific Pacific social risk and protective factors can assist in developing innovative practice strategies to address criminogenic and recidivist offending behaviour.
- Promoting good policy responses to resource effective rehabilitative responses within the legal system is an important approach to youth justice.
- Utilising Pacific models of practice will also ensure a culturally appropriate and holistic approach.

Introduction to youth justice and Pacific youth

Youth offending is a tricky area of work that requires a nuanced and pragmatic understanding of the complexities that lead to such occurrences happening in and across society. This includes the notion of criminogenic factors that may underpin the reasons why people offend. However, such complexities become even more complicated when trying to understand offending in the context of other social and welfare needs, alongside other areas of diversity and its differences. For example, the notion of Pacific youth offending is made complex when first trying to understand Pacific youth in the context of their stage of psychological development, whilst then trying to position this perspective alongside their socio-economic context, their familial structures, their use of traditional Pacific languages and their commitment to faith/spirituality further paired with other Pacific cultural practices across their own ethnic community. Too often society simply sees youth crime through a moral lens, viewing this as selfish actions of the offender rather than the possible reasons as to why people offend, which raises the need to create a fair and just response to deterring such behaviour and activity. In this chapter, such complexities will be explored, with a view to highlighting the importance of understanding the many factors that may lead to Pacific youth offending across Oceania, including the Pacific Islands, and the diaspora residing in places like New Zealand and Australia.

The role of ecological systems and social capital

The old adage, *context is everything*, rings true for Pacific youth offending. The need to gain a deeper insight and understanding as to why Pacific young people may offend is the underlying key to also create effective responses to counteracting the concerns that lead to such problematic occurrences. Generally, the role of *ecological systems theory* in social work is part of this quest to gain a deeper understanding, where a person is understood in their context of their family, community and other factors they interact with. There is a relationship that occurs between the way in which the various parts of a system may operate, and the ability to gain benefits within a system provides insight into how well the system works. There are multiple levels to a system, with varying levels of impact that may also occur. For example, if an education system requires students to learn in a certain manner and places certain expectations on parents to support and also assist in facilitating a particular approach to learning at home is not understood, then a child's ability to engage in learning may be affected. The same is true with the role of the health care system. If there is a limited understanding and inability to access services to support wellbeing, then this will affect an individual's ability to gain support for positive health outcomes. Similarly, society is made up of multiple systems, and the way in which one learns to interact and access its benefits is also influenced by the notion of *social capital*. The idea of social capital reflects the ability of an individual to successfully navigate and interact with other people and places and to acquire skills, knowledge, behaviours and attitudes that will assist in gaining positive life outcomes. However, how can one navigate and gain positive skills for life if the systems they are interacting with aren't set up to assist in this process? It is within this space that such answers need to be found, especially when looking at Pacific youth offending. And again, with this approach in mind, it is important to understand youth offending in the context of whether it is occurring in the Pacific Islands or across places like New Zealand and Australia. It is also within these settings that possible solutions can be found, and we will continue to look at this across research, policy and practice.

Research across youth justice

Offending trends

While Māori are over-represented at every stage of the New Zealand criminal justice system, comprising over 50% of the total prison population, Pacific

Islanders are third behind Pākehā, making up 12% of the total prison population (Statistics New Zealand, 2017).

New Zealand is second to the United States for the highest rate of imprisonment per head of population in the OECD (Organisation for Economic Co-operation and Development) (Maxwell, 2011). Pacific Islanders make up 8.9% of the total crime apprehension, which is relatively high considering that Pacific Islanders make up only 7.4% of the total New Zealand population (Statistics New Zealand, 2017). It is estimated that the rate of cases involving Pacific young people is growing, with crime apprehension approximately twice the rate than that of European young people and half the rate of Māori (ibid). According to Ioane, Lambie and Percival (2016), *A Comparison of Pacific, Māori, and European Violent Youth Offenders in New Zealand* study of Pacific youth offenders highlighted common factors such as they were "born in Aotearoa, raised in low socio-economic deprivation areas and that their exposure and involvement in family violence was high" (p. 25).

Emerging studies across Oceania reveal that the Pacific youth offending problem is no longer just a New Zealand issue. In Australia, Pacific youth offenders feature significantly in the growing gang culture and are involved in numerous violent offending (Ravulo, 2016; White, 2013). Given that New Zealand has the largest Pacific population outside of the Pacific Islands, Nakhid (2012) argues that the importance of addressing Pacific Island youth offending and the strategies implemented in New Zealand are of ongoing international interest. The social impact of Pacific youth offending reveals social exclusion. Pacific people in New Zealand experience inequality in that they are over-represented in most of the negative statistics, especially a low socio-economic status (Ioane & Lambie, 2016). They are at the wrong end of the negative crime statistics such as being significantly over-represented as perpetrators and victims of family violence. As a result, they are less likely to report family violence or to access support services (Ioane, Lambie & Percival, 2013; Ioane et al., 2016; Kaloto, 2003; New Zealand Ministry of Justice, 1999; New Zealand Ministry of Social Development, 2002).

Australia and New Zealand's Pacific Island population is made up of a large percentage of youth aged 15 years or younger (Ioane et al., 2013; Ravulo, 2015). Further studies suggest that youth offenders are social outcasts because of a lack of structural and systemic opportunities to support them in education, employment, housing and constructive pro-social activities (Barry & McNeill, 2009). A further discourse outlines the dearth of scholarly literature on Pacific youth offending to also assist in gaining a better insight on the causes of such concerns. Ioane et al. (2016) point out that more research is needed given there is growing disparity of social, economic and educational risk factors for Pacific youth and by not actioning this may see a continuation of this over-representation in negative statistics. In saying this, there needs to be more research in this area by Pacific researchers themselves, with an emphasis on the use of Pacific models and methodology in mainstream institutions (Ioane, 2017). Acknowledging these offending trends can then further assist in being able to unpack the reasons why such issues occur. The need to then explore from an ecological or bigger picture point of view can then assist in creating a deeper understanding of the criminogenic factors; that is, factors that lead to offending and the possible solutions to counteract.

Risk and protective factors

Therefore, with the above in mind, this yields broader conversations around the social and welfare needs of Pacific youth offenders, with previous research undertaken on the risk and protective factors that may exist. Developed by Jioji Ravulo (2009), Table 8.1 outlines the possible factors associated across three areas: individual and family, peer and community and education, employment and training. Each of the three domains provide context for areas that need to be understood (firstly the risks) to then be counteracted through possible solutions (protective factors).

In essence, risk factors are areas that need to be first understood in the context of what is happening for the individual Pacific young person, whilst also developing a richer perspective on how their family, peers, community and their interaction with education, employment and training occurs. To assist in creating developmental response, where this context is further understood, risk and protective factors are then provided as a platform to create innovative, engaging and effective responses that deter offending behaviour, whilst also evolving systemic practices towards social inclusion and justice. This may also influence service delivery models and its provision, including case management, counselling and community development approaches.

Policy and its implications

According to Scott (2003), the estimated cost to society of the 1% of teenagers who ended up in prison was around $3 million each over their lifespan. The impact of crime on the economy is also significant, with the cost of crime in general increasing considerably from $1.7 billion in 2009 to $3.4 billion in 2010 (Maxwell, 2011). The significance of these figures is that although youth offenders make up a small proportion of society, it accounts for a high cost to society through an ever-increasing rate of youth offending (Fergusson, Horwood & Lynskey, 1994, as cited in Kiro, 2009). While there is no specific data on the cost of Pacific youth offending, most studies illustrate high costs through the disproportion of Pacific youth offenders. Furthermore, studies reveal the growing cost of youth offending relates to increased spending in incarceration as opposed to rehabilitative or preventative strategies (Barry & McNeill, 2009). However, international and domestic studies indicate that fiscally incarceration is not the solution and so effective strategies are crucial in building positive futures for at-risk youth and the communities that sustain them (Cunneen, White & Richards, 2016).

TABLE 8.1 Pacific youth risk & protective factors

Domain	Risk factors	Protective factors
Individual & family	• Communal negative alcohol usage from parents • Excessive violent (physical and verbal) behaviour within family home and community • Lack of verbal reasoning • Lack of access to privately owned, registered vehicles • Lack of knowledge about accessing Social Security benefits • Overcrowding in family homes • Parental low level of secondary education • Lack of access to Proof of Identification • Older sibling involved in crime • High-level care given by older siblings to younger siblings	• Cultural inclusiveness within family home • Enhanced understanding of Western systems (education, health, legal, community) for both young person and parents • Development of verbal communication skills • Positive attitudes towards lifelong learning
Peer & community	• Negative involvement with police • Excessive/binge usage of alcohol and marijuana • Misinterpretation of presenting behaviours by professional legal settings • Lack of rapport with non-Pacific adults in community setting • High level of infringement notices and fines • First offence being of a serious indictable nature • Negative peer group association through organised gangs • Lack of consistent attendance at court due to no parental support • Conflicting ideologies developed between Western & Pacific culture • Legal conditions that contradict family relations • Active enrolment in school during court proceedings • Inconsistent approach and access to physical and mental health care services	• Active involvement in sporting commitments • Genuine involvement in spiritual and faith-based activities • Enhanced relationship with police who appreciate Pacific culture • Enhanced relationship with teachers who appreciate Pacific culture • Participation in cultural activities across community • Strong sense of community participation reinforced by Pacific relatives also living in Australia

(Continued)

TABLE 8.1 (Continued)

Domain	Risk factors	Protective factors
Education, employment & training	• Lack of educational resources • Parents undertaking more than one full-time job to maintain financial stability • Early school leaving (pre-Year 10) • Misinterpretation of presenting behaviours by professionals in education • Lack of training and advancement for parents predominantly employed in low-skilled labour force	• Positive association and awareness of educational institutions for both young person & parents • Access to vocational training courses for both young person and parents • Consistent attendance at school • Access to support and training materials in assisting educational placement • Continuation of schooling beyond middle years • Focus and desire during adolescence to undertake vocational interest

The last youth offending strategy tabled by the New Zealand government was the Youth offending strategy that was launched by the Ministry of Social Development in 2002 (New Zealand Ministry of Social Development, 2002). The strategy outlined the importance of addressing youth offending, especially Māori and Pacific Islander youth offending, and the government commitment to this problem. Unfortunately, the majority of the programmes that were funded to address this problem, especially Māori and Pacific Islander specific programmes, no longer exist today.

In Australia, the ongoing development of culturally relevant practices are being considered by the New South Wales (NSW) Department of Justice, who convene a Pacific Steering Group made up of Pacific community members to further assist burgeoning strategies. This approach was first instigated through a NSW Partnership with Pacific Communities in the early 2000s – which formally dissolved on completion of a funding-specific initiative to combat Pacific youth crime (ARTD Consultants, 2007). However, as this is an ongoing concern raised by NSW Police, and the Pacific community, the need to implement such strategies via the NSW Department of Justice remains on the agenda.

More broadly across the Pacific region, the need to ensure policies are developed to assist government resourcing of programmes that support the proper legal processes to occur is also important. As seen in the case study following, this includes Island states and territories ensuring timely responses can occur, and other social and welfare support and programmes are embedded as part of the systemic response to rehabilitation.

CASE STUDY 8.1: YOUNG OFFENDERS IN FIJI

Suva is the capital of Fiji and the most densely populated area in the country. It is also one of the largest Pacific Island cities. Crime is a growing concern, particularly theft and the violence that sometimes accompanies it. Pita* works with young men who entered the justice system between the ages of 15–20 years. Generally, young men's first offences are aggravated robbery. Generally, they are repeat offenders.

As part of his work, Pita provides life coaching to these young men. There are times when he provides them temporary shelter and acts as surety for bail hearings. All of the young men Pita works with no longer live with their own families. They were either kicked out of the family or are ashamed and afraid to go back into the family fold.

Some of the experiences the young men have had include the use of violence by police officers;

> Police officers are often threatening to me even though I didn't do it. They physically abuse me even step on me with their boots. The Crime department who often charge also deal with me threateningly

unsatisfactory prison conditions;

> Prison wardens unfairly treat us in prison. Bedding that we are given is often old, torn and worn out. Food [dhal] that we eat inside is just liquid. At times when in prison and it is our court attendance dates, we often remind wardens of our clothes – could it be cleaned but these fall on deaf ears. They do not allow us to wash our own civilian clothes

and an unfair court system;

> Justice system is not fair. Inefficiency within the court's as there is a great backlog of cases. Sometimes we request speed trial but due to this backlog we are told that it cannot. Speed trials are requested because sometimes we are unjustly charged with other crimes when our cases are pending due to delayed court proceedings. The police sometimes when they cannot solve other crimes in town they tend to blame us because we are well known to them and we are often seen in town areas. But the perpetrators come from outside of town.

The young men suggest that:

- *Police should speak to us non-threateningly and respect our answers. Don't coerce us to say what they want to hear.*
- *If the police can have prosecution knowledge in the station. If they know that the cases won't be able to stand in court because of lack of evidence then they should not charge the person at all.*

> - *The police need to be trained in other techniques of acquiring information from people instead of being abusive.*
>
> Pita argues that sometimes the authorities are lax in the execution of their duties, especially during court days:
>
> > One young person that I was coaching was treated unfairly when upon the calling of his case at Court # 3, he was still locked up in the holding cell below. The officers were slow in bringing the prisoners to court when their cases were called. Resulting in their being taken back to the remand centre. I had actually turned up to be a surety for him so he could be bailed. It was a sad case to see the young people neglected and treated unfairly in this manner by the system.
>
> *The social worker's name has been changed to protect the confidentiality of the young people he works with.

Practice for a Pacific purpose

A multidisciplinary approach to youth justice is needed as its impact affects families and communities. The scrutiny of youth offending in the media is generally negative and the public view of social workers in this field can at times be less forgiving. There are two Pacific models that may assist social workers in working with Pacific youth offenders. The *Fonofale* model is a Pan Pacific practice model that is widely used in the health and social sectors (Meo-Sewabu, 2015; Pulotu-Endemann, 2001). The second Pacific model is the *Talanoa model*, developed in 2006 by Timote Vaioleti, and is based on Pacific oral traditions (Vaioleti, 2006). It is important that as a practitioner the young person and their family are felt listened to and are reassured that they have the power to speak freely and without interruption. This process is also where Pacific oral traditions underpin the intervention approach and actions.

In a Western social work context, this process of communication would be the social practitioner's reflective lens, which is important in social work supervision (Connolly, Harms & Maidment, 2018). However, Farrelly and Nabobo-Baba (2014) provide the Pacific understanding of the term *talanoa*, which is the process by which Pacific people can offload freely much like "chewing the fat" or debriefing. In working with Pacific youth and families, making connections or building rapport is far more important than highlighting the rationale of one's role or policies that dictate the reasons a client must engage the process. Research by Mooney (2010) highlighted the importance of social workers building rapport with Māori youth based on a Māori worldview that embodies physical, spiritual and cultural connections. Such Māori worldview elements may parallel with the

Pacific worldview and especially the Fonofale model (Pulotu-Endemann, 2001). With this in view, the second recommended Pacific approach, the *Fonofale model* is a holistic framework of wellbeing in the shape of a *fale* (house) with interconnected and interdependent life domains represented by different parts of the *fale*, which parallel a Pacific person's values and beliefs. The roof of the *fale* represents culture, the overarching value and belief systems of Pacific Island families. According to Pulotu-Endemann (2001), the dynamics of Pacific people adapting to New Zealand culture places them on a continuum where they are either Westernised or more inclined towards traditional Pacific culture. According to Anae (1998), the struggle of cultural identity experienced by New Zealand born Pacific people is a plausible explanation of why some turn to crime or gangs to try to fit in.

Therefore, developing a cultural understanding of the individual and family may assist in counteracting significant social and welfare needs, whilst positively engaging the young person and their support in the possible process of change beyond offending.

PRACTICE EXAMPLE 8.1

Developing and Implementing a Case Management Model for Young People with Complex Needs (Mission Australia & Ravulo, 2009): A specific toolkit was developed to assist community workers, educators and justice officers to better engage with young offenders, including those from Pacific communities. Informed by empirical research, this document provides a framework to understand the process of working effectively in the context of case management and includes a suite of tools that practically assist in engaging young people.

Conclusion

Overall, the idea of working effectively with Pacific young offenders is generally multifaceted, which requires a multi-lens and multi-systemic approach. This includes understanding the context in which the individual is positioned within their immediate environment with their family, peers and wider community, whilst also gaining insight into how they interact with the various social systems that surround them. In turn, individual capacity and capital can be built to further assist the young person and their family to successfully navigate the complexities they may experience from their social and welfare needs, whilst negotiating the support needed from others. This includes the role of social workers to also challenge and reshape the way in which statutory agencies interact with such young people, including the creation of collaboratively approaching the position of the offender in a broader context and understanding.

Rather than seeing young offenders as problematic individuals, social workers should be versed in understanding the many contexts in which this person exists, including their cultural values and beliefs that should also be part of the bigger solution and strategy to a fair and equitable approach across achieving youth justice.

> **REFLECTIVE QUESTIONS**
>
> 1. What broader societal factors do you need to consider when developing a case plan with a Pacific young offender?
> 2. What strategies could be developed to assist other stakeholders to develop a better working relationship with Pacific young people and their families?
> 3. What additional resources could be developed by the government to help counteract youth offending?
> 4. What role does traditional cultural knowledges and its practice play in supporting positive participation for all young people in their own communities?

References

Anae, M. (1998). *FOFOA-I-VAO-'ESE: The identity journey of NZ-born Samoans*. University of Auckland.
ARTD Consultants. (2007). *Evaluation of the NSW Youth Partnership with Pacific Communities 2005–2007 – Final report to the Implementation Committee*. Sydney, Australia: Author.
Barry, M. & McNeill, F. (2009). *Youth offending and youth justice*. London: Jessica Kingsley Publishers.
Connolly, M., Harms, L. & Maidment, J. (2018). *Social work: Contexts and practice* (4th ed.). South Melbourne, Australia: Oxford University Press.
Cunneen, C., White, R. & Richards, K. (2016). *Juvenile justice: Youth and crime in Australia* (5th ed.). South Melbourne, Australia: Oxford University Press.
Farrelly, T. & Nabobo-Baba, U. (2014). Talanoa as empathic apprenticeship. *Asia Pacific Viewpoint*, 55(3), 319–330.
Ioane, J. (2017). Talanoa with Pasifika youth and their families. *New Zealand Journal of Psychology*, 46(3), 38–45.
Ioane, J. & Lambie, I. (2016). Pacific youth and violent offending in Aotearoa New Zealand. *New Zealand Journal of Psychology*, 45(3), 23–29.
Ioane, J., Lambie, I. & Percival, T. (2013). A review of the literature on Pacific Island youth offending in New Zealand. *Aggression and Violent Behavior*, 18(4), 426–433.
Ioane, J., Lambie, I. & Percival, T. (2016). A comparison of Pacific, Maori and European violent youth offenders in New Zealand. *International Journal of Offender Therapy and Comparative Criminology*, 60(6), 657–674. https://doi.org/10.1016/j.avb.2013.05.002
Kaloto, A. (2003). *The needs of Pacific Peoples when they are victims of crime*. Wellington, New Zealand: Ministry of Justice.

Kiro, C. (2009). Children parenting and education: Addressing the causes of offending. *Policy Quarterly, 5*(2), 19–23.

Maxwell, G. (2011). *The cost of crime: Towards fiscal responsibility.* Wellington, New Zealand: Milne Printers Ltd.

Meo-Sewabu, L. D. (2015). *The cultural constructs of health and wellbeing amongst Marama iTaukei in a Fijian village in Lau and in a transnational Fijian community in Whanganui, Aotearoa.* Palmerston North, New Zealand: Massey University.

Mission Australia & Ravulo, J. (2009). *Developing and implementing a case management model for young people with complex needs.* Sydney, Australia. Retrieved from http://nla.gov.au/nla.obj-254917404/view

Mooney, H. (2010). *The value of rapport in Rangatahi Maori mental health: A Maori social work perspective.* Massey University, New Zealand.

Nakhid, C. (2012). 'Which side of the bridge to safety?' How young Pacific Islanders in New Zealand view their South Auckland community. *Kotuitui: New Zealand Journal of Social Sciences Online, 7*(1), 14–25. https://doi.org/10.1080/1177083X.2012.670652

New Zealand Ministry of Justice. (1999). *Responses to offending by Maori and Pacific peoples: A 1999 crime annual review.* Wellington, New Zealand. Retrieved from www.justice.govt.nz/publications/publications-archived/1999/responses-to-crime-annual-review-1999/responses-to-offending-by-maori-and-pacific-peoples

New Zealand Ministry of Social Development. (2002). *Youth Offending Strategy: Preventing and reducing offending by children and youth people.* Wellington, New Zealand: Author.

Pulotu-Endemann, F. K. (2001). Fonofale model of health. *Pacific Models for Health Promotion,* 7.

Ravulo, J. (2009). *The development of anti-social behaviour in Pacific youth.* Sydney, Australia: University of Western Sydney.

Ravulo, J. (2015). *Pacific communities in Australia.* Sydney, Australia. Retrieved from www.westernsydney.edu.au/__data/assets/pdf_file/0006/923361/SSP5680_Pacific_Communities_in_Aust_FA_LR.pdf

Ravulo, J. (2016). Pacific youth offending within an Australian context. *Youth Justice, 16*(1), 34–48. https://doi.org/10.1177/1473225415584983

Scott, G. (2003). *The economic benefits of rehabilitating chronic adolescent anti-social males.* Auckland, New Zealand: Youth Horizons Trust.

Statistics New Zealand. (2017). *Statistics New Zealand Prison population.* Wellington, New Zealand. Retrieved from http://archive.stats.govt.nz/browse_for_stats/snapshots-of-nz/yearbook/society/crime/corrections.aspx

Vaioleti, T. M. (2006). Talanoa research methodology: A developing position on Pacific Research. *Waikato Journal of Education, 12*(1), 21–34.

White, R. (2013). *Youth Gangs, Violence and Social Respect – Exploring the Nature of Provocations and Punch-Ups.* London: Palgrave Macmillan.

Suggested further readings/websites

For case law and legislation for 20 Pacific Island countries see http://www.paclii.org/

Comprehensive website outlining legal information for each state and territory in Australia is made available from the *LAWSTUFF – know your rights*: www.lawstuff.org.au

In New Zealand, a helpful website is *YouthLaw – Free Legal help throughout Aotearoa*: http://youthlaw.co.nz

9
APPLYING CULTURALLY APPROPRIATE APPROACHES WHEN WORKING WITH PACIFIC ADULT OFFENDERS

Jioji Ravulo and Julia Ioane

Key points
- Adult offending is multifaceted and complex, requiring a more nuanced and exploratory approach to understanding its causes and possible solutions.
- Australian and New Zealand policies on deporting offenders have had an impact on Pacific people and their ability to access resources and adequate support regionally.
- Culturally inclusive practices are occurring across the region, with a view to promoting a meaningful approach to addressing personal issues through family and community support.

Introduction of field and social work theory

Across the globe, there are various ways in which offending behaviour is understood. Generally speaking, Western-informed societies prescribe to a classical view where people are seen to offend within the context of making a "rational choice" (Loughran et al., 2016). For example, someone who decides to steal a car did so with a possible rational reason to sell this for financial gain. As a result, the person if caught should be punished for making such a rational choice with a view to deter them from undertaking this type of behaviour in the future. Over time, this creates a black and white perspective on crime, with adages developed like "you do the crime, you do the time" and "crime doesn't pay". This dominant way of thinking, also known as discourse, then perpetuates an ongoing societal view that people should be punished for making such bad decisions. Governments then create legislation and its accompanying policies to create legal systems that may include various forms of punishment, which generally includes subjecting such people to incarceration, locking them away for a determined amount of time in prisons. Certain crime will then carry a certain amount of time or level of retribution the person needs to "pay" for such behaviour.

However, more and more research, including that informed by disciplines like social work and psychology, question the role of such punitive measures on the individuals that are subjected to such punishments. At the same time, the notion that people always exercise "rational choice" to commit a crime has also been challenged with the view that there are complex reasons as to why people may offend, and how we should then create other possible solutions to deter this from happening again. Various crime prevention strategies are created to support the negative and harmful impact towards victims of crime, however, the need to also promote adequate resources, research and approaches to counteract the social issues that people who offend may be experiencing is also just as important. This chapter will explore the context of adult offending across the Pacific, with a view to promoting inclusive strategies in working effectively with Pacific adults who offend. Pacific cultural perspectives on offending and various approaches will be profiled to show a shared and collaborative view between cultural ways of doing things and how this may be aligned with contemporary perspectives and practices. More so, the chapter will strive to challenge the way in which we understand the structural inequalities that may exist in society that in turn perpetuate circumstances that lead to people committing crime across the region.

Structural violence and its impact on societal systems

Structural violence is a concept that acknowledges the creation of certain injustices that may occur when certain dominant discourses, or ways of doing things, are developed and maintained at the detriment of privileging one group over others. The distribution of resources across society is also skewed, where those that have access to resources continue to develop structures to maintain their power and influence, whilst those that don't have access to such resources, or positions of influence, are not heard and continue to be marginalised and discounted (Hosken, 2016). In social work, we perceive society not as a homogenous entity, but rather as a group of systems that are developed to assist in the functionality of society and to help the various communities, families and individuals within. An example is the education system. Resources are developed and distributed in accordance with what is believed to be correct at the top level, and people are then mandated to undertake certain expectations established within. But what happens if the system leaves you behind as a result of not creating practice and policy that is based on meeting your diverse needs? This could be on the basis of your learning style or your access to other resources to help you learn, like computers and Wi-Fi access. In turn, this would deter your ability to engage in formal education, which may limit your employment options as you may not have the necessary skills to acquire and maintain sustainable employment. Over time, this may then create issues with being able to earn money, which then jeopardises the ability to access finances to support other areas of need including stable accommodation, food supplies and positive recreational activities. And this all occurred from your inability to be catered for within an education system designed by those with power and influence. This is an example of structural violence – where systems and other areas of society have created a lack of opportunity, now relegating such people to areas of disadvantage, including poverty.

Unfortunately for some, instead of creating pro-social behaviours and attitudes to function in society, these forms of structural violence may create anti-social behaviours and patterns of thinking that leads to offending and crime. This includes the use of alcohol and other drugs, including illicit substances, which may lead to exasperation of poor mental health and wellbeing. Therefore, society is faced with various challenges to create systems that are not geared towards perpetuating such forms of violence, but rather one that is inclusive of diversity and its difference. It is within this context that adult offending can be further understood, and the way in which we treat such social concerns should be multifaceted and explored. This includes being able to see the perpetrator in the context of their personal, cultural and structural needs. Such perspectives mirror the anti-oppressive approach, also evident in social work thinking. Over time, a re-shifting may occur where practice approaches with individuals and families work hand in hand with community resources and groups that are supported by systems and structures that truly deal with the causes of offending. Therefore, the notion of good practice, policy and research that pervades these areas of the personal, cultural and structural can work together, subsequently addressing the micro, meso and macro perspective of society.

Wider and broader context of Pacific offending and its consequences

In the context of Pacific adult offending, there are also diverse perspectives at play too. In the Pacific Islands, anti-social behaviour has been dealt with across various settings – from within the traditional village location based on roles and responsibilities to ensure harmony amongst the community, to the more urbanised settings where statutory systems including police, courts and prison come into effect. There is a need to consider both a traditional approach – where village elders and leaders oversee the consequences given to individuals or groups who have disrupted the expected coherence found in village life and where cultural values and perspectives are included and utilised to restore a positive communal environment – and to ensure justice is provided. On the other hand, the role of the perceived contemporary practices of arresting people, bringing them before a court to be sentenced by magistrates instituted by the government and then possibly incarcerating them within a punitive setting is also very real and part of reality across the region. Such tension needs to be further understood and a collaborative or shared approach between the two is something various Pacific Islands are doing to ensure traditional and contemporary practices are upheld.

Across the diaspora in places like Australia and Aotearoa New Zealand (hereafter referred to as Aotearoa, the indigenous word for New Zealand), Pacific adults, similar to their juvenile counterparts, are over-represented in the adult correction system. In Aotearoa, the most up to date and available data on Pacific offenders report that 12% of all prisoners are of Pacific ethnicity (Department of Corrections NZ, 2015). Given the diversity of the Pacific, just over 40% of Pacific offenders are Samoan followed by Cook Island/Rarotonga and Tongan, with just over half born in Aotearoa. Pacific prisoners tend to be younger when compared to non-Pacific prisoners, however, half of Pacific prisoners receive sentences of over 5 years compared to 45% of non-Pacific prisoners.

Current data provided by the Department of Corrections in Aotearoa show that the largest offences committed by Pacific people are violent offences (37%), followed by sexual offences (9.5%) (P. Johnston, personal communication, 4 September 2018). Similarly, Pacific youth offenders are also over-represented in their violent offending (Ioane & Lambie, 2016). Such trends have at times challenged the perception of Pacific people as being positive contributors to society, as they may be perceived and labelled as anti-social due to the nature of the crimes committed by such Pacific people. Stereotypes of this nature can then further perpetuate issues of personal, cultural and structural violence and the detriment of the community as a whole. This negative perception is further reinforced by the many Pacific community members residing in low socio-economic areas, for example, greater Western Sydney, where the largest urbanised cohort of Pacific people reside in Australia, followed by areas of South Brisbane (Ravulo, 2015). Similarly, the largest Pacific population in Aotearoa reside in South Auckland, known also for its similarly low socio-economic settings; characterised by high rates of poverty, large public housing estates, issues with educational attainment and concerns with unemployment or low-skilled employment (Policing Development Group Counties Manukau District, 2007). Once again, these social and welfare issues may generally parallel with the notion of *criminogenic factors* that relate to characteristics that lead to anti-social behaviour, including crime.

The next three sections on research, policy and legislation and practice will further highlight the need to employ a bigger and broader perspective on adult offending discussed earlier, profiling social work perspectives and approaches in working effectively across the community.

Historical and cultural contexts in contemporary settings

The need to include Indigenous perspectives in the way in which legal systems deal with such offenders further reiterates a call to challenge the ongoing over-representation of such people in the adult system. Horrifically, the over-representation of Aboriginal and Torres Strait Islander peoples in the correction systems across all states and territories in Australia highlights such concern, which has also been mirrored by Māori in New Zealand and iTaukei in Fiji.

Tracing the historical records of crime in New Zealand from 1852–1919, Bull (2004) suggests that racist practices in instituting a westernised and *white is right* approach to Māori has resulted in systems being created that now continue to perpetuate and uphold such methods in modern day Aotearoa, including issues of inter-generational trauma and oppression as a result of being involved in such racist institutional approaches. Naylor (2011) suggests that due to the colonial influences of ensuring westernised standards are upheld, westernised legal practices and perspectives create an ongoing stigma for the offender, rather than promote true rehabilitation for the reason why people may offend. As a result, offenders are marred with a lifelong label that may deter their ability to truly succeed in life beyond the crime committed, perpetuating a cycle of recidivist offending behaviour and perspectives. A need to create a better insight and understanding by such legal practices is required, including the promotion of ongoing funding and resourcing of early intervention and prevention and the development of meaningful approaches to restorative justice. The need to also nuance legal systems that also cater to other diverse perspectives, including those based on gender, are also important. Women from a Pacific background who offend may find it more difficult to adjust to life after incarceration (Brown, 2006), and the need to promote cultural perspectives which includes roles and responsibilities within this cultural context is also vital to positive success post-incarceration.

Restorative justice is part of the broader conversation undertaken across research in the region, where offenders and the wider community are brought together to ensure justice is provided to all. In this context, many Pacific-related perspectives on the collective and communal approach underpinning traditional perspectives are paralleled. In a seminal piece written by Maxwell and Hayes (2006), they suggest restorative justice works well with Pacific people due to this notion of shared responsibility and providing offenders, their victims and the local community with a view to reconcile and ensure responsibility is undertaken by the offender in lieu of their crime. This includes the Te Whanau Awhina model, where Maori offenders are brought onto a marae alongside support people and elders who focus on reconciling the person with the wider community. Therefore, through restorative justice approaches, such research suggests that the use of traditional practices is meaningfully included in this way where Pacific people are given the scope to navigate and negotiate their experience in the formal legal systems in a more culturally nuanced manner.

Additionally, Whitehead and Roffee (2016) suggest the need to also meaningfully ensure the right balance between offending types and retribution occurs when integrating traditional perspective with westernised practices. For example, the way in which victims of child sexual abuse are involved in the justice process undertaken in customary restorative practice in rural villages across the Pacific can be tricky. The lack of resourcing that may exist to assist the child to receive appropriate rehabilitation beyond the reconciliation that may occur between the offender and the village community needs to be further considered.

Deportation policy and its impacts on the Pacific

Despite its history as a penal colony where convicts were settled from Great Britain and Ireland in the late 1700s and early 1800s, Australia has now positioned itself with a strong commitment to deport offenders that have ethnic ties elsewhere. Through the establishment of the Deportation of Non-Citizen Criminals scheme (The Parliament of the Commonwealth of Australia, 1998), specific policy and its related legislation has been created to send convicted residents back to their country of origin; even if they settled in Australia as a child, and/or have no actual family back in the country they are to be deported to. This includes the growing number of Pacific people residing in Australia who after spending time in custody are being deported directly upon release from gaol via first being placed in an immigration detention whilst the order is being finalised and executed. It is within this practice that many Pacific people are being divided from their family living in Australia and being sent back to New Zealand or the various Pacific Island states, with further restrictions that they aren't able to ever return. Such levels of scrutiny continue to perpetuate concerns for Pacific people who may return into the region with no immediate family support, including accommodation, access to finances and other means to reintegrate back into life after incarceration. This can and does have a follow-on effect as such Pacific people may resort to areas of anti-social behaviour and crime to survive, which in turn leads to possible reoffending and incarceration. For others, they may be able to develop stronger cultural and kinship ties, enabling positive pathways to inclusion across society. Nonetheless, this policy from Australia is having an impact on Pacific families, both in the diaspora and the wider region, and such impacts should be taken into consideration when working with Pacific adult offenders who have been deported.

In Aotearoa, there appears to be some confusion with the number of Pacific people deported back to the Pacific Islands. Corrections data shows that a decline in the number deported from nine in 2010 to one in 2017 (P. Johnston, personal communication, 9 October 2018). However, this requires further exploration due to the number of police escorts of prisoners to the Pacific Islands in the last year. Of note, over 33% of offences that led to a deportation were due to violence (37%), followed by sexual offences (21%). One of the biggest issues following deportation is the lack of transition planning from one country to the next. When a prisoner is returned to Samoa from Aotearoa, they are escorted by members of police from Aotearoa and released to police in Samoa. It is unclear whether proper transition essentially occurs between the police as a prisoner can be released to no one upon arrival and is therefore expected to fend for themselves. The challenge is to seek out the appropriate support for the prisoner pending on their circumstances and ensure there is clear communication to the country receiving the prisoner. There needs to be a legislative approach within Justice to ensure that when Pacific prisoners are deported to their country or island of origin (usually a Pacific Island), it does not inadvertently inherit the issues with that prisoner. This can create a resourcing issue that the island is unable to manage appropriately, which has potential to cause harm to the community or village. In some way, there needs to be a targeted approach to collaboratively working towards a transition plan that is well thought out, considered and mitigates risk of the offender towards themselves and to the community or village to which they are deported to. There is a responsibility within policy to ensure that the health, wellbeing and safety of the deportee and community is upheld.

Culturally related and relevant practice

Through the opportunity to employ restorative justice approaches and its practices within indigenous cultures like those found across the Pacific, we believe structural violence can be alleviated. In accordance with Maxwell (2008) on crossing cultural boundaries and indigenous contexts, there are several key reasons restorative justice works. We have mapped and quoted these key areas alongside the three areas of an anti-oppressive approach evident in social work approaches, as outlined in Table 9.1. In essence, each level of oppression is being addressed, with the view that other areas still need to be understood and dealt with. Additionally, it is important that restorative justice is utilised where appropriate, which includes ensuring victims are not subjected to further concerns as a result of this process. However, overall, this bigger picture approach may yield and position systems to be more humanly responsive to the needs of the offender, rather than perpetuate cycles of disadvantages and disorder.

Holistic practices that adequately address the way in which individuals are understood in the context of their personal issues and how this sits within a cultural and structural context is important. This includes embedding case management and counselling approaches that address and counteract criminogenic factors including the conventional need to promote motivation to access

TABLE 9.1 Promoting restorative justice with adults across Pacific social work

Anti-oppressive approach (level of oppression)	Maxwell (2008) important elements to restorative justice
Structural	"evokes a past when the clan, the tribe, the village or the community gathered to resolve among themselves the wrongs that could otherwise threaten their cohesion" (p. 93)
Cultural	"emphasise not only taking responsibility and repairing harm but also treating people with respect, and working toward reconciliation and healing" (p. 94)
Personal	"it does not need to be constrained within a universal format but can be allowed to adapt to the customs of the people who are participating in it" (p. 94)

vocational training and other related skills that will assist with job readiness leading to successful employment. However, for Pacific people, it is more than acquiring a job to support themselves. Conversations within a case management or counselling context with Pacific adult offenders need to also incorporate a bigger, communal perspective. In westernised approaches, case management and counselling focuses on the individual and their own understanding of self, and how this can relate to others. But within a Pacific perspective, the need for an individual to position their own view of self is greatly dependent on others; including parents and significant others such as partners, grandparents, aunties and uncles, cousins and peers. By having the individual person understand their own actions on others in this bigger system may further promote a customary view of accountability to others and may also support the scope for offenders to position their offending away from an individual ambition to a wider impact.

Group work can also have a positive impact on working with adult offenders. In a group work context, providing a scope for individuals to discuss and share their situation and concerns associated with wellbeing and other key areas can be highly therapeutic and effective. In most cases, being able to base these sessions within a gender-specific context (a group for men, a group for women, etc.) can enable participants to feel more comfortable, and respectively communicate in a relational manner. Operating from a strength-based approach can also assist in the facilitation of conversations that share both challenges and successes, with a view to highlight what skills participants can utilise to reach individual and family goals. Also, apart from being a safe space to share, this approach is also underpinned by the Pacific notion of *Talanoa*, where people enter into a collective dialogue that promotes positive space and place.

CASE STUDY 9.1: AOTEAROA

The s27 of the Sentencing Act (2002) acknowledges the use of a cultural assessment to address (though not limited to) the cultural background of the offender, the way in which their background may have contributed to the offence and how support from whānau and community may be relevant to prevent offending. Anecdotally, it is understood that there is a growing awareness for s27 reports from the District Court to be directed. More recently, case law was made with the admission of a culturally based counterintuitive assessment in High Court highlighting the growing awareness within the Justice sector in Aotearoa to understand the worldview of indigenous and ethnic minority communities that include Pacific (R v Taimo HC Auckland CRI-2016-085-2938, 21 September 2018, Moore J). The inclusion of cultural assessments and understanding the diversity of worldviews is crucial to formulating targeted assessments and interventions to minimise and eliminate the risk of recidivism and working towards better outcomes for Pacific adult offenders. Additionally, a specialised rehabilitation programme called *Saili Matagi* is being implemented in the prisons, adapted for Pacific men to work towards a non-offending lifestyle. It draws on Pacific cultural principles using a "proverbial language approach" to transfer cultural values, beliefs and concepts into a therapeutic programme to reduce recidivism and improve outcomes for Pacific offenders (King & Bourke, 2018).

CASE STUDY 9.2: SAMOA

The *matai* (chiefly) system in the prison has provided a unique relationship between prison staff and prisons (Office of the Ombudsman Samoa & Samoa National Human Rights Institute, 2015). A review of the Ombudsman reported that due to this relationship, outcomes have improved (Samoa Observer, 2016). The *matai* system provides the only form of counselling to prisons, which has benefits to prisoners. However, it is still noted that prisoners still need to receive appropriate professional counselling. Another example of where the *matai* system is in operation is due to staff working together with matais in the prison to prevent escaping from prison. When a prisoner is re-captured, they will be seen by a council of matais. There is a matai from the cell and they will provide *talanoa* with the prisoner before they are returned to the punishment cell. However, there is a growing need for further resources to maintain the matai system as a culturally appropriate mechanism for effective management and containment of prisoners, leading to better outcomes post-sentencing.

CASE STUDY 9.3: FIJI

The implementation of the *Yellow Ribbon* programme (Fiji Corrections Service, 2014) across prison locations in Fiji is promoting developing meaningful vocational and life skills for inmates before returning back into their own communities. The programme also strives to promote positive messages across schools and the wider community on providing adult offenders with a second chance post-release, demystifying certain stereotypes and labels on adult offenders, which can then mar positive re-integration into society. This approach reflects a broader cultural consideration on the offender still being seen as a valued part of the family and village where they originate, whilst esteeming their collective contribution to the wider community.

From a macro perspective, promoting scope for legal organisations working with Pacific people to also work within a culturally relevant manner is just as important. This includes the utilisation of cultural awareness training through workshops, or access to reports and other scholarly material that helps better enhance practice within these spaces to occur. Workers from both Pacific and non-Pacific backgrounds can further enhance their effectiveness by learning how to ensure cultural safety is part of the foundation in which practice, policy and research occurs, whilst also implementing the notion of cultural harmony. Such approaches ensure that workers are critically reflective about their interactions and work with the client in a collaborative manner, rather than reinforcing power relationships instated by statutory bodies.

Conclusion

Pacific adult offending is complex in nature and should be understood and approached in a similar manner. That is, rather than discounting the many social and welfare needs associated with the individual that offends, we need to be more multifaceted in creating systemic responses that meaningfully engages and makes a difference. This includes implementing service models and provisions that effectively position the offender in their wider cultural and societal context to ensure a collective approach is undertaken that resonates with the worldview of Pacific people. It would also be an innovative solution to work towards a judicial system that reflects the offending population it serves, with a significant proportion of indigenous and ethnic minority judiciary promoting policy that informs institutional and organisational practice that are culturally appropriate and enhance research that promotes the meeting of customary restorative practices within contemporary legal settings.

> **REFLECTIVE QUESTIONS**
>
> 1. Having an understanding of the social and welfare issues and needs of people who offend is important. Discuss why this is the case, and why such perspectives may shape good research, policy and practice.
> 2. How would you practically ensure the use of traditional perspectives are used when undertaking case management support to adult offenders? How does this then apply to the broader family and community?

References

Brown, M. (2006). Gender, ethnicity, and offending over the life course: Women's pathways to prison in the Aloha State. *Critical Criminology*, *14*(2), 137–158. https://doi.org/10.1007/s10612-006-9001-5

Bull, S. (2004). "The land of murder, cannibalism, and all kinds of atrocious crimes?" Maori and crime in New Zealand, 1853–1919. *British Journal of Criminology, 44*(4), 496–519. https://doi.org/10.1093/bjc/azh029

Department of Corrections NZ. (2015). *Pacific offenders*. Wellington, New Zealand. Retrieved from www.corrections.govt.nz/resources/research_and_statistics/topic_series_reports/pacific_offenders_topic_series_report.html

Fiji Corrections Service. (2014). *About Yellow Ribbon*. Retrieved from www.corrections.org.fj/pages.cfm/yellow-ribbon/about-yellow-ribbon.html

Hosken, N. (2016). Social work, class and the structural violence of poverty. In B. Pease, S. Goldingay, N. Hosken & S. Nipperess (Eds.), *Doing critical social work – Transformative practices for social justice* (1st ed., pp. 104–118). Sydney, Australia: Allen & Unwin.

Ioane, J., & Lambie, I. (2016). Pacific youth and violent offending in Aotearoa New Zealand. *New Zealand Journal of Psychology, 45*(3), 23–29.

Johnston, P. (2018, September 4). Personal communication via email.

Johnston, P. (2018, October 9). Personal communication via email.

King, L., & Bourke, S. (2018). A review of the Saili Matagi Programme for male Pacifica prisoners. *Practice: The New Zealand Corrections Journal, 5*(2), 1–5.

Loughran, T. A., Paternoster, R., Chalfin, A., & Wilson, T. (2016). Can rational choice be considered a general theory of crime? Evidence from individual-level panel data. *Criminology, 54*(1), 86–112. https://doi.org/10.1111/1745-9125.12097

Maxwell, G. (2008). Crossing cultural boundaries: Implementing restorative justice in international and indigenous contexts. *Sociology of Crime Law and Deviance, 11*, 81–95. https://doi.org/10.1016/S1521-6136(08)00410-7

Maxwell, G., & Hayes, H. (2006). Restorative justice developments in the Pacific region: A comprehensive survey. *Contemporary Justice Review, 9*(2), 127–154. https://doi.org/10.1080/10282580600784929

Naylor, B. (2011). Criminal records and rehabilitation in Australia. *European Journal of Probation, 3*(1), 79–96. https://doi.org/10.1177/206622031100300107

Office of the Ombudsman Samoa & Samoa National Human Rights Institute. (2015). *For Samoa, by Samoa: State of the human rights report*. Apia: Author.

Policing Development Group Counties Manukau District. (2007). *Counties Manukau police district environmental scan*. Auckland, New Zealand: New Zealand Police.

Ravulo, J. (2015). *Pacific communities in Australia*. Sydney, Australia. Retrieved from www.westernsydney.edu.au/__data/assets/pdf_file/0006/923361/SSP5680_Pacific_Communities_in_Aust_FA_LR.pdf

Samoa Observer. (2016, April). Ombudsman inspects Tafa'igata Prison. *Samoa Observer*. Retrieved from www.samoaobserver.ws/en/03_04_2016/local/4467/Ombudsman-inspects-Tafa'igata-Prison.htm

The Parliament of the Commonwealth of Australia. (1998). *Deportation of non-citizen criminals*. Canberra, Australia: Commonwealth of Australia.

Whitehead, J., & Roffee, J. (2016). Child sexual abuse in Fiji: Authority, risk factors and responses. *Current Issues in Criminal Justice, 27*(3), 1–7. Retrieved from http://search.informit.com.au/documentSummary;dn=950302287;res=IELAPA

Suggested further readings/websites

The Pacific Islands Legal Information Institute (PacLII) facilitated by The University of the South Pacific profiles legislation across 20 Pacific Island countries: www.paclii.org/

Ministry of Justice in New Zealand provides an overview on the various sections of the legal system across Aotearoa: www.justice.govt.nz/

Legal Aid in Australia is available across each state and territory and may be available for free based on certain situations and circumstances. www.australia.gov.au/content/legal-aid

10

COMMUNITY DEVELOPMENT

Connecting research, policy and practice in Pacific communities

Dunstan Lawihin, Wheturangi Walsh-Tapiata and Kesaia Vasutoga

Key points

- Community development approaches within the Pacific need to be culturally relevant.
- Community development defines a large part of social work in the Pacific.
- Principles of practice define community development and include: having a vision; indigenous frameworks; bottom-up development; community ownership and participation; the personal is political; process orientation and social change.

Introduction

> *Ehara taku toa i te toa takitahi, engari he toa takitini.*
> My strength is not mine alone, but the strength of the collective.
> *(Māori proverb)*

Community development practice in the Pacific is a communal process aligning with collectivist values in traditional communities. However, development policies, research and community practice models draw significantly on western ideas which often marginalise local experiences, knowledge and wisdom.

This chapter challenges the Pacific sector to build culturally relevant community knowledge, policy frameworks and practice approaches. Colonialism pervades much of the Pacific and what we do in social work and community work. In order to speak back, in order to claim our voice in this setting, we need to value our local knowledges and practices. We need to recognise the paramountcy of communal culture and collective spirit to family and community wellbeing. Without the knowledge and understanding of local cultures, community development interventions and research approaches can lead to insensitivity to local cultures and values and to unfavourable outcomes in Pacific communities, perpetuating colonial practices believed to be the only way. Community development is more synergistic with the communities of the Pacific than professional social work is, given its collective-community approach rather than an individualised approach.

This chapter looks at what community development is and means in the context of the Pacific. Differing understandings may lead to tensions in the knowledge, policy, research and practice terrains, particularly as we consider what our respective traditional communities understand to be community development from our localised contexts. The inclusion of local knowledge and lived experiences acknowledges the place and culture in which community development functions. Knowledge of diverse community contexts – both internal Pacific and international diversity – is necessary for practitioners.

The three writers of this chapter traverse three nations of Oceania. Dunstan comes from Papua New Guinea, Kesa is from Fiji and Wheturangi is from Aotearoa New Zealand. We all work in our communities and utilise a community development framework which derives from our cultural contexts. Understanding cultural contexts is core to practice and central to any consideration of knowledge, policy and research around community development. Know your community and know yourself in the context of your community.

Definitions of community development

Many terms that describe work in community, such as "community organising" and "community planning", are used to describe a directive, top-down approach to working in communities (Munford & Walsh-Tapiata, 2001). "Community development" focuses on a process of working alongside, directed by the community, around issues that the community have identified (Munford & Walsh-Tapiata, 2001, p. 5). Ife (2016) describes community development as,

> a vision of a future society based on the principles of ecology, social justice, post-Enlightenment and Indigenous world views, achievable through an empowerment approach to the development of community in which human needs are met primarily at community level.
>
> (p. 123)

Ife believes that in a world of increasing instability where many solutions at a global level appear to only make things worse, development at a community level provides a more viable and sustainable solution to localised issues. Similarly, The International Association of Community Development (IACD) (2016) states:

> [Community Development] ... promotes participative democracy, sustainable development, rights, economic opportunity, equality and social

justice, through the organisation, education and empowerment of people within their communities, whether these be of locality, identity or interest, in urban and rural settings.

(p. 8)

The UN (undated) defines community development as a process by which the efforts of the people themselves combine with government efforts to improve the economic, social and cultural conditions of communities and integrate these communities into the life of the nation and enable them to contribute to national progress. This definition anchors on two main principles of development practice.

i. Participation of people in efforts to improve their living standards with as much reliance on their own initiatives; and,
ii. The provision of technical and relevant other services that encourage community initiative, self-help and mutual help to make them more effective.

Therefore, community development is a process that involves community members coming together and taking collective actions to solve common problems. This definition, thus, indicates that community development is an approach of strengthening civil society by prioritising the actions of communities and their perspectives in the development of social, economic and environmental policy.

The shared goal, therefore, of community development is to achieve a better life for the whole community through collective action, albeit the issues and the practice will be different to each community and will require a localised community response. Community development starts from and with the community and thus it occurs from "below" or from the "inside" going out. It is not just an activity, it is not just a job, it is a process and it requires a certain mindset which informs the way in which one works. It is a politically contested practice where a range of people can adopt the term but sometimes with very different interpretations. The United Nations Development Program (UNDP) (2016, p. 10), whose work is prevalent in the Pacific and emphasises that community development is a "process of doing", works together to identify and develop economic and social opportunities, skills, leadership, confidence and community bonds for the advancement of the whole community wellbeing.

The Pacific Community (2015) has a vision for the Pacific region which builds on community development when they state, "Our Pacific vision is for a region of peace, harmony, security, social inclusion and prosperity, so that all Pacific people can lead free, healthy and productive lives" (p. 2). The ambition, therefore, of the community is to progress the quality of its people's lives and increase their participation in decision making to achieve long-term improvements. In writing about Tongan community development, Mafile'o (2005) emphasises the need to work together for the collective good. Munford and

Walsh-Tapiata (2006, p. 98) agree with Mafile'o in acknowledging culture as a foundation to any work that occurs in their communities.

Within the Pacific space, definitions of community development, informed by their own knowing, are less definitive and the default has been to resort to Western models. This can create some uncertainty around the implementation of community development in local communities. The Pacific needs to consider what community development looks like for them based on collectiveness and communalism. Principles of practice might help to inform this.

Principles of practice

One of the distinguishing features about community development are its values and principles which inform practice. They are not a "how to do it" or about imposing one's own agenda or scheme of things on others. They develop organically from the community, dependent on the cultural, economic, social and political context of that community (Ife, 2016, p. 177). They should, however, inform your practice and your mind-set, characterising a view about how society works and a vision of how it can work. These guide ones' daily practice by helping to analyse and identify how situations that communities face can be transformed. Pearce and Kay (2005) define values as what we believe in and the principles that underpin and guide what we do. Across different Pacific communities, the following principles could help to inform community development practice. Additionally, others could be added that are particular to your community.

Having a vision

It is important for community or community workers to build a vision for the future or of how a situation can be changed for the betterment of the collective. It can be as broad as social justice for all, or it can be focused to align with a goal that the community wishes to achieve for themselves (Munford and Walsh-Tapiata, 2006, pp. 99–101): "A vision helps to form a basis for finding a direction, for achieving positive change and sustaining this change". The indigenous people of Aotearoa interpret vision as *moemoea*, articulating their dreams through stories from the past that help to inform the present and the future. It connects the generations and helps to sustain the people in particularly hard and challenging times. Similarly, traditional village communities in Papua New Guinea (PNG) often draw from the past using the family-tree approach to secure the future of its younger members, evident in the land tenure system.

Indigenous frameworks

Specific to the Pacific will be the need to include the needs, the cultural worldview and the practices of indigenous populations and local ethnic groups.

The Pacific is fraught with nations, with agencies and with people who come from the outside, who bring a different view of the world and who attempt to impose this thinking and practice on communities in an almost benevolent way. As the indigenous movement grows around the world, there is a recognition that indigenous frameworks should be used in indigenous development. For some Pacific nations still firmly imbedded in their cultural communities, this principle may be questioned, but the influence of colonialism and the need to speak back from an indigenous knowing is critically important. Nabobo-Baba (2006) talks about the importance of examining and discussing indigenous epistemology as this allows the insider to tell their own story and link to their cultural practices and traditions.

Indigenous frameworks, therefore, have to be core to community development within the Pacific context. One such example is that of starting from the "telling my story – known to the unknown" in facilitating community empowerment training for local community development officers in PNG. Such an approach to facilitation and learning enables a free and comfortable space for indigenous participants to share their own lived experiences and knowledge in an empowering manner prior to learning about contemporary, often foreign concepts and principles. Another example in Aotearoa New Zealand has been the battle for the revival of the indigenous language and culture through the development of Kohanga Reo (immersion in early childhood education), which is now firmly embedded in the education system of the country and has been extended to primary school, college and tertiary education.

Bottom-up development

Understanding the local context, local knowledge, resources, energies and capacities are central to development, planning and practice in communities. The views of community members and community leadership are integral in defining the development path of specific communities as this ensures that the visions, expectations and plans of the community are captured. The best practice in PNG and potentially other parts of the Pacific confirms that a bottom-up development approach is effective and achieves best results when it is participatory, democratic, inclusive and gender balanced (UNDP, 2016). In many instances, outside influences have in fact hindered rather than helped a given situation. An example in Fiji is a bilateral aid El Nino project that focused on providing efficient and safe irrigation systems for farming. The project was known to have worked in some Asian countries and involved generating water by using a pair of wheels to cycle and add pressure. However, as the average weight of a Fijian farmer was heavier than an Asian farmer, most of the pumps broke after a few uses. This is an example of how donor communities can perceive community development in Pacific countries to be homogeneous to the Asia-Pacific diaspora. This is a perspective that must be re-imagined.

Community issues require community workers to work alongside the community as local knowledge and practices are a central tenet to the change process. Sanga et al. (2005, p. 12) confirm that Pacific peoples are relational where extended family and heritages are the way that they live. They are close knit and guard their identities passionately. Community development at all levels needs to have this awareness rather than outsiders coming in and imposing their thinking in this space. Insider contribution, for Maori by Maori, is increasingly prioritised in the tribal development of Aotearoa New Zealand. Similarly, the localisation programmes have been undertaken by the PNG public service since the 1970s; such approaches to development encourage local community members to lead and offer core contributions of change in their community for Pacific people by Pacific people.

Community ownership-community participation

Communities prosper when they develop their own solutions to their own problems. By working collaboratively and collectively they then claim community ownership. It is important therefore that everyone participates in the process, with all key stakeholders committing to practice and to the ability to compromise along with continual action-reflection to ensure that goals are being met.

Enabling local people to be involved in community development projects is important whatever their varying degrees of capabilities and challenges, even if only in a small way. The combination of everyone together contributes towards the whole of advancing communities. Some people may need additional support to overcome the barriers they face and effective participation in development will include poverty, disability, age, culture and ethnicity, geography and other circumstances that may be seen to marginalise people. Valuing diversity in and from the community ensures that all contributions are embraced, where all community members are heard and participate in the processes that affect their lives. Given the collective nature of many Pacific communities, this should be attainable, although the hierarchical nature of these communities might also provide a challenge. The community development worker needs to recognise that many people and agencies can contribute to achieving community development goals at personal, family, community and societal levels.

Ample examples exist of community ownership and participation drawing on Pacific indigenous strengths. Service charters applied in PNG Correctional Services and the Village Courts and Land Mediation Services encourage community and key stakeholder participation in the management and delivery of the services. Collective decision-making in the Maori culture is core to its development aspirations – the whole community is working as one – *mahi tahi*. Similarly, the Fiji's world view of community and social welfare is evident through the *solesolevaki* tradition. The *solesolevaki* tradition is grounded on the ideals of reciprocity and communalism. *Solesolevaki* is evident, for example, in co-operative stores which have been sustained for 40–50 years in some parts of Fiji, generating revenue which is shared annually amongst tribes and clans, including children.

The personal is political

Working in this space requires a mindset where you are regularly challenging structural oppression by looking at issues of social justice, equality/fairness and solidarity of human rights. It is important to value fairness along with justice thereby striving to reduce inequities and to uphold human rights that seek to ensure access, equity, participation and legal protection for all. As Ife (2016, pp. 183–184) states:

> The links between the personal and the political, the individual and the structural, or private troubles and public issues, are essential components of community development...as they offer a critical step in consciousness-raising, in empowerment and in developing a plan of action.

Empowerment is a central tenet of social justice and human rights and therefore people of the community need to be at the core of the development process. Community development workers play a significant role in facilitating the process of empowerment by aiming to increase the power of those disadvantaged populations in our communities whereby they gain more control of decision-making and action over their life situations.

Political decisions in many parts of PNG have become a family and personal thing and are made along the lines of maintaining power and control as well as soliciting support – "the wantok system." This system is popular in Melanesia and when applied appropriately, can lead to securing and achieving social security objectives for families and members of the community subject to conditions of vulnerability (Lawihin, 2017). The case in New Zealand is more a legislative requirement where tribes are now going through the Waitangi Tribunal process to investigate their own history and reclaim their identities and birth rights. These indigenous frameworks are useful for integration into contemporary democratic principles and ensure culturally relevant development practice.

Process oriented

Being process oriented is an important aspect of community development, albeit there is often a tension between process and outcome. Learning to trust the process can be challenging for people, particularly if they pragmatically want to move directly to outcomes. Process can be equally challenging if you still do not have an outcome that you are working towards. Time is a critical factor in ensuring that process is allowed to occur. Pacific communities can have a different understanding of time and the importance of ensuring that the correct cultural protocols are observed, which need to be taken into account in any community development initiative. There may be times when you need to take steps backwards in order to ensure the process has been covered thoroughly in order to move towards and to achieve the vision of the community.

Community development workers of Pacific origin focus on the process and believe that this increases the chances of achieving quality development outcomes. Some local non-government organisations (NGOs) in PNG have utilised facilitation as the main method to demonstrate that community development is process oriented. This process begins with a request, to story, to agreement, intervention, monitoring and evaluation (Interchurch Organization for Development Cooperation [ICCO] & German Development service [DED], 2004), a process that is similar to that for community development (Roberts, 1979). The request and agreement signify engaging in consensus decision-making, a key feature in other Pacific communities.

Social change

Community development is about understanding how oppressive structures can be challenged and transformed; therefore, ultimately it is important that positive social change occurs for the group. The combined efforts and local social capital are key to achieving social change. The sharing of knowledge between groups enables people/communities to learn from each other in terms of what has worked or not worked.

The challenge is to maintain any gains made so that this becomes an expected outcome of any initiative. For community and with community is critical to social change that is long term and sustainable. Pacific communities are known for their cultural and ritualistic ceremonies showing community success and solidarity. For Pacific Island communities, it is important that social changes and improvements are celebrated to instil a sense of inclusiveness, ownership and a baseline for long term sustainability.

Implications for community development

Community development is foundational and largely defines social work in the Pacific. Given its focus on a community-led and self-help development approach, community development is relevant to all communities of the Pacific. Isolation, low income-earning opportunities and poor access to services have been identified as common issues in the Pacific, affecting rural areas and in particular in PNG and Melanesia (UNDP, 2016). Respective Pacific Island state governments have responded appropriately through community-oriented policies that encourage community-led development and bottom-up planning. PNG presents a good example through its decentralisation policies and the Integrated Community Development Policy focusing on empowering communities through the establishment of District Development Authorities (UNDP, 2016) and Community Development Learning Centres. This government approach has been applauded as culturally relevant and addresses real community challenges.

However, in the Pacific, there are less definitive connections between community development and social work, thus there is some level of uncertainty as to whether or not community development is the overarching home that hosts social work practice. To treat community development as homogenous is erroneous. The multiple levels of community systems and cultural protocols need to be unpacked, analysed and understood by educators, practitioners and policy makers prior to engaging with Pacific communities – a dynamic space requiring high levels of flexibility.

Although community development and social work are distinctly defined in the Aotearoa New Zealand context, key principles of human service practice such as social justice, human rights and empowerment are common denominators that exist in both practice fields. While international definitions of social work and community development are clear, regional and national definitions need to be developed that fit the Pacific context. Given the slight variations in Pacific cultures in specific national contexts, the definition needs to be contextual, yet flexible to be applicable in diverse contexts of practice.

Pacific community development is too often external-led. This situation is evidence of neo-colonialism in the Pacific where the "powerful" West uses economic, technological and cultural conditioning to enforce their development models and laws on our people (Narokobi, 1983), yet encapsulated in "attractive" international development and foreign policy agenda. This makes it difficult to achieve the goals of community-led development and active local participation, subsequently undermining the principles of community empowerment and sustainable development.

There is a need for Pacific-Indigenous social entrepreneurship to underpin community development and promote self-determination and to resource Pacific community-led change – based on cultural strengths. Being a self-help approach to development, community development cannot occur in communities that depend highly on external support. Valuing local culture, resources and skills to drive self-help development reduces high dependency on external aid. External support, though, has driven community development in the Pacific, but it has implications on lasting progress and long-term sustainability. This is because the supply of expertise and resources is external and does not guarantee insider control and ownership, limiting any prospects for sustainable development.

Indigenous Pacific professionals must therefore be seen to be leading the research and development of culturally appropriate development models in the Pacific. Effective and relevant community-led development is one that is inclusive by focusing on supporting all members of the community, with special emphasis on children, women, elderly and people living with disabilities. Whilst research on Pacific-Indigenous methodologies for community development is at its infancy stage, local researchers and academics have a critical role to play in building community development knowledge and relevant development models in the Pacific for the Pacific.

In some Pacific countries, such as the Melanesian region, the mere absence and the feebleness of national social and community work bodies have contributed to that lack of a clear and strong definition of community development and social work. Thus, there is a heavy reliance on international definitions and knowledge and research published in Australian and New Zealand literature. Generally, community development and social work are emerging fields of research and policy yet there is a long history of application within the Pacific. Amidst minimal research knowledge and general practice, both social work and community development are struggling to be recognised as a profession. In countries such as Fiji, community development in institutions such as the University of the South Pacific (USP) recognises it as a methodology in social work practice. On the other hand, institutions such as the Australia Pacific Technical College (APTC) and Auckland Institute of Technology (AUT) run community development programmes which are distinct and separate from social work. Government agencies, churches, corporations and NGOs have been involved in the practice of community development over many years.

The significance of community development in the Pacific

Community development from an ecological perspective focuses on sustainable development principles and practices that need to be integrated in order to be consistent with the current global, regional and national development needs and visions of respective Pacific nations. Community development is best placed to develop a nation "from below" and contribute to the achievement of national development visions and UN's Global Sustainable Development Goals. It is a development approach that works when development is "community-led" and is benefiting the whole society from the local to the national, regional and global levels. In communities, community development seeks to challenge conditions which create vulnerability and disadvantage but more significantly, UNDP (2016) confirms that community development empowers the "hands that knows their need" (p. 11). Empowering communities builds their confidence to identify, talk about and prioritise their needs and take actions to address them. This further helps communities to develop a sense of community ownership and accomplishment when there is improvement and change in their livelihoods. These accomplishments are often celebrated through significant levels of community success and togetherness (UNDP, 2016). Some of these benefits have been evident in the UNDP Community-Led Millennium Development Goal Acceleration Pilot Project (CLMAP) in PNG. UNDP and its partners in this project identified some benefits of community development:

- Conflict resolution and reduced conflicts between clans
- Increased cooperation between inter-community, faith and clan
- Youth engagement, skills development and reduced anti-social behaviour
- Women empowerment, challenging traditional roles
- Access to education

- Strong sense of ownership and pride
- Increased transparency in local level decision making
- Civil engagement
- It leads to further development (success breeds success)

This practical evidence suggests that community development strengthens peoples' confidence, skills, ownership and knowledge about what it takes to drive development at local village and ward levels. In view of national development, community development enables better diversification of the economy, redistribution of resources and power of decision making to those provinces and districts in need. Subsequently, there is increased level of resilience among communities and people, a natural tenet of Pacific Island communities.

Thus, community development in this text is defined as a practice-based discipline informed by research that promotes and enhances social, economic and ecological wellbeing of communities, whether these be of locality, identity or interest, in urban and rural settings, and recognising the comprehensive cultural systems within every setting prior to acting. Pacific communities are rooted on a common vision and a common journey. This is where community development can thrive because it is a collective practice (Aimers & Walker, 2013). A collective practice suggests that in order to achieve community development goals, cultivating a shared vision and building trust among community members is critical. Therefore, our Pacific working definition of community development is a process where community members come together to take collective action and generate solutions to common problems. Community wellbeing (economic, social, environmental and cultural) often evolves from this type of collective action being taken at a grassroots level.

Conclusion

Community development as presented in this chapter is a small yet beginning and evolving contribution from the Pacific perspective. This contribution is mostly from Fiji, New Zealand and Papua New Guinea; however, references are made to a broader Pacific regional context acknowledging collective cultural commonalities and specific internal socio-structural variations. The significance of this chapter is that we attempted for the first time to define and fit community development both as an approach and activity in the context of Pacific Island communities in relation to the global community.

With lack of research and knowledge base that is of Pacific origin, community development of Western origin has dominated community development practice and knowledge in the Pacific. There is clear acknowledgement of these Western contributions. The chapter has highlighted some aspects that undermine valuable cultural assets that have been the strength and foundation of Pacific Island communities and clearly articulates the need for Pacific communities to be the drivers of their own approach to community development.

References

Aimers, J. & Walker, P. (2013). (Eds.) *Community development: Insights for practice in Aotearoa New Zealand*. Auckland, New Zealand: Dunmore Publishing.

Ife, J. (2016). *Community development in an uncertain world: Vision, analysis and practice* (2nd ed.). Melbourne, Australia: Cambridge University Press.

Interchurch Organization for Development Cooperation [ICCO] & German Development service [DED] (2004). Organization in focus: A Papua New Guinean approach to organization development, Interchurch Organization for Development Cooperation.

Lawihin, D. (2017). *Building a culturally relevant social work curriculum in Papua New Guinea: Connecting the local and global in field education.* Unpublished Master of Social Work (research) Thesis, Monash University.

Mafile'o, T. (2005). Community development: A Tongan perspective. In M. Nash, R. Munford and K. O'Donoghue (Eds.). *Social work theory in action*. London: Jessica Kingsley Publishers.

Munford, R. & Walsh-Tapiata, W. (2001). *Strategies for change: Community development in Aotearoa/New Zealand* (3rd ed.). Palmerston North, New Zealand: School of Social Policy and Social Work.

Munford, R. & Walsh-Tapiata, W. (2006). Community development: Working in the bicultural context of Aotearoa New Zealand. *Community Development Journal, 41*(4), 426–442. doi:10.1093/cdj/bsl025

Nabobo-Baba, U. (2006). *Knowing and learning: An Indigenous Fijian approach*. Suva, Fiji: Institute of Pacific Studies, University of the South Pacific.

Narokobi, B. (1983). *Life and leadership in Melanesia*. Institute of Pacific Studies, University of South Pacific and University of Papua New Guinea.

Pacific Community (2015). *Pacific Community Strategic Plan 2016–2020. Sustainable Pacific development through science, knowledge and innovation*, www.spc.int/resource-centrePacific Community, Noumea.

Pearce, J. and Kay, A. (2005). *Social accounting and auditing: The manual*, Liverpool, United Kingdom: Social Audit Network

Roberts, H. (1979). *Community development: Learning and action*, Toronto, Canada: University of Toronto Press.

Sanga, K., Chu, C., Hall, C. & Crowl, L. (2005). (Eds.) *Re-thinking aid relationships in Pacific education*. Wellington, New Zealand: He Parekereke, Institute for Research and Development in Maori and Pacific Education, Victoria University, and Suva, Fiji: Institute of Education, University of the South Pacific.

The International Association of Community Development (IACD). (2016). IACD – About. *Whanake: The Pacific Journal of Community Development, 2*(2), 3–12.

United Nations Development Program (UNDP). (2016). Community Development in Papua New Guinea "Yumi Olgeta Wok Wantaim": A Good Practice Manual. Empowering and Supporting Communities to Grow and Prosper. United Nations Development Programme in Papua New Guinea.

11

UNDERSTANDING THE VĀ FOR SOCIAL WORK ENGAGEMENT WITH PACIFIC WOMEN AND CHILDREN

Selina Ledoux-Taua'aletoa

Key points

- Pacific people venerate the collective, defining themselves through relationships or *Vā*. When the *Vā* is both respected and acknowledged social workers can develop a point of reference for developing therapeutic relationships and interventions for women and children.
- The *Fonofale* model aligns well with the Ecological Systems Theory (EST) and can inform practice, once professionals have created a *Vā* of respect and honour.
- Approaching from a strengths based approach (SBA) will strengthen the *Vā* and encourage positive successful engagement that provides fertile ground for positive sustainable outcomes.

Introduction

This chapter discusses a relationship or *vā* perspective for social work practice with Pacific women and children, whether in their country of origin or in the diaspora. Proverbs and cultural practices affirming the importance of women and children are presented as points of reference and connection when working with Pacific families. The chapter looks at policies that promote wellbeing and practice approaches that enhance the strengths within Pacific families. The case study in this chapter invites you to reflect on how one might embed appropriate cultural approaches to enhance wellbeing for children and women.

Pacific perspectives on the value of women and children

Successfully engaging with Pacific communities and families requires appropriate approaches. Proverbs can guide professionals engaging with Pacific families and communities, providing points of connection to inherent values and principles. *E fōfō e le alamea le alamea* (Anon, Sāmoan Proverb) is a Sāmoan fishing proverb that literally translated means "the crown-of thorns starfish can heal its own doing". When you are stung by the crown-of thorns starfish, turn the starfish upside down and its sponge-like feet will reabsorb its toxins. This proverb denotes that there is power within people to find solutions that create opportunities for healing (Autagavaia, M. June 15, 2015 personal communication).

Many Pacific traditions and proverbs provide insight into the value of children and women. For Tongans, the *fahu* is an excellent indication on the sanctity and importance allotted to women (Helu, 1995). The *fahu* is the role given to the oldest sister of a generation. The role is unique to the Tongan culture and is a role of great importance for Tongan families. The *fahu* is afforded respect by her male sibling's children. As an example, when the niece or nephew to the *fahu* gets married, the *fahu* will sit at the head table and receive traditional gifts from the family. The *fahu* role includes the naming of the children of her male sibling. The *fahu* are, however, expected to conform to a higher standard of behaviour than her sibling, being respectful and appropriate at all times, taking on, for want of a better description, the role of matriarch for the *kāinga* (family). This is not withstanding that parents are still given due respect as the parents and leaders of the *kāinga*. The *fahu* needs to have an excellent understanding of *anga fakatonga* (Tongan way) in order to provide good and appropriate advice and direction to the *kāinga* when needed (Sofele, K. October 4, 2018 personal communication).

Fijians have the *vasu*, the child of the sister to a Fijian male. These child/ren are spoilt by their maternal uncles and their families (Tuifagalele, Q. September 28, 2018 personal communication). Another Fijian practice is the vacating of space. This can be misinterpreted as avoidance, rather, it is a show of respect where a brother may leave the room or space when their female sibling enters, the brother in essence is giving the space to his sister. A sister will do the same for her male sibling. You may see this behaviour occurring when a child or young person leaves the room when adults enter, the behaviour a manifestation of respect, the child or young person is giving the adults the space (Tuifagalele, Q. September 28, 2018 personal communication). These Fijian practices affirm the importance of a respectful sibling relationship, adult and child/ren relationships and the value attributed to women.

In the Niuean culture, children are served their meals first, they are also the first priority in grooming. These seemingly small everyday practices are an indication of the priority attributed to children. This is the behavioural manifestation of the importance of children and the adult role to provide service and protection (Talima, A. & Moala, S. August 21, 2018 personal communication).

The following are Sāmoan and Tokelauan proverbs denoting that the nurturing of children is done through words. There is no Sāmoan proverb encouraging physical harm against children for any reason, inclusive of discipline.

> '*O tama a tagata e fafaga i upu ma tala, a'o tama a manu e fafaga i fuga o la'au*'. (young birds are fed with the blossoms of trees whereas the children of people are fed with words).
>
> *(Anon, Sāmoan Proverb)*

> '*Ko te tama a te manu e fafaga i nā ika, ko te tama a te tino e fafaga i nā kupu*'. (Rather than use the *halu* [cane] on children it is much wiser to use words of reason).
>
> *(Anon, Tokelauan Proverb)*

The *wharenui* (big house or the main meeting house on the *marae*) of *Tangatawhenua* (people of the land or the indigenous people of Aotearoa [New Zealand]) is also known as *te whare tangata* (the house of people) or the womb of women that holds people. The door of *te whare nui* or *te whare tangata* symbolises the vagina. It can only be entered by invitation and with respect. The space within *te whare tangata* is sacred ; conversation and conduct are mediated by protocols and rules that foster unity and harmony (Wallace, E. May 25, 2018 personal communication).

Impact of colonisation on Pacific communities should be considered when engaging with Pacific women and children. Culture has been used as an excuse or a mask for the ill-treatment and abuse of women and children. However, the Pacific traditions and values indicate that violence within the family was not condoned (New Zealand Ministry of Social Development, 2012). Culture is dynamic, and Pacific cultures have changed significantly over time in response to many different factors inclusive of colonisation (Thaman, 2003).

Violence has become misunderstood as being part of Pacific culture; this reinforces the idea of how dynamic culture is. It is therefore conceivable that as cultures continue to evolve, people and communities can make conscious efforts to move away from violence and towards an existence that respects and cherishes all family members, particularly women and children.

> *E fōfō e le alamea le alamea.*
>
> *(Anon, Samoan Proverb)*

There are values held in common by many of the Pacific nations that promote and enhance the wellbeing of individual family members and the family as a collective. Values such as reciprocity, *tapu* (sacred) relationships, genealogical knowledge, language and a sense of belonging are examples (New Zealand Ministry of Social Development, 2012, p. 5). We need to begin to understand sacred relationships in terms of the *vā* (Anae, 2016).

Vā literally means space between people in both Samoan and Tongan. Maori use the word *wā* to describe the same concept. The *vā/wā* is the space in which people relate to each other, whether that is between family members or between professionals and the communities that they work alongside of (Anae, 2016). Each of the aforementioned examples of behaviour within the *'āiga/kāinga/ whānau*/family provide a glimpse of how important the nurturing and maintaining of respectful relationship are evidenced. *Vā* can be used as a point of reference to elicit behaviour that is respectful between *'āiga/kāinga/whānau*/family/ community members and professionals.

Policy

Policies relating to women and children differ across the region. The United Nations (UN) Convention for the Rights of the Child (CRC) recognises children have rights to wellbeing, and all 22 countries and territories ratified the CRC. Pacific countries and territories provide protection through tradition. CRC ratification acknowledges how removed *āiga/kāinga/whanau*/family/communities are from traditions.

Most Pacific countries and territories developed legislation and policies upholding rights of women and children. Levels at which policies and legislation are imbedded in social work differs between countries and territories. In 2006, a Pacific Regional Framework involving Fiji, Vanuatu, Sāmoa, Kiribati, Solomon Islands, UNICEF and AusAID was developed. The Pacific Regional Framework provided strategic direction for child protection interventions within participating countries.

The Convention on the Elimination of All Forms of Discrimination Against Women (CEDAW), adopted by the UN in 1979, provides a platform for realising equality between sexes. It promotes equal access for women in politics, education, health and employment. There has been positive movement, however, there is still work to be done:

> more than 60% of women in some Pacific countries have experienced physical or sexual abuse. Across the Pacific, men outnumber women in paid employment outside the agricultural sector by approximately two to one. Women make just 4% of parliamentarians in the Pacific (lowest rate in the world), compared with a global average of around 21%.
> *(Pacific Community & United Nations, 2016)*

World Health Organisation (WHO) (2018) statistics indicate globally that suicide was the third leading cause of death in 15–19 year olds in 2016, the second highest cause of death for females in the age bracket. The WHO identified risk factors to adolescent mental-wellness: poverty, violence, forced migration, substance use, chronic illness, harsh parenting, bullying, sexual violence, early pregnancy, forced marriages, discriminated group status (World Health

Organisation, 2018). Adolescence is a vulnerable time where young people are trying to define themselves.

Inadequate representation of women and children in politics and policy design, combined with vulnerability, requires social workers to engage in ways that promote positive outcomes. Providing women and children a voice by working at a micro level directly with women and children and the macro level through policy (Brofenbrenner, 1990) addresses this. Engaging theories, models and practices relevant to Pacific communities should be considered in engagement and assessment to promote positive outcomes.

Theory, models and practice

Ecological Systems Theory (EST) aligns with Pacific cultures and values (Bronfenbrenner, 1990; Nash, Munford & O'Donoghue, 2005; Cumming & Allen, 2017). Models such as *Fonofale* (Endemann-Pulotu, 2001) sit naturally under the EST umbrella, acknowledging the importance of understanding people in context, focusing on both the individual and their environment. EST provides a platform for assessing wellbeing holistically, understanding people from points of interdependence and relatedness (McMahon, 1996). Effective engagement with women and children requires understanding cultural values and roles.

> Through you, my being is contextually meaningful and whole. Through myself, you are given primacy in light of our collective identity and places of belonging (*fa'asinomaga*), our genealogical lineage (*tupuaga*), and our roles, responsibilities and heritage (*tofiga*).
>
> (Tamasese, Peteru & Waldegrave, 1997, p. 13)

Endemann-Pulotu (2001) developed the *Fonofale* framework/assessment tool, which can be used in working alongside Pacific women and children. Pulotu-Endemann used a meeting house analogy with a roof, four poles and foundation. The four *pou* (poles) represent physical, mental, spiritual and other. Spirituality, commonly overlooked by Western models, holds significance for Pacific people. Spiritual wellbeing understood simply is aligning behaviour with values. Values held may be religious or founded in tradition – reciprocity is a value held by most Pacific people and ensures that support given is received. It is a value held prior to Christianity and remains an integral value to most Pacific cultures. The word reciprocity does not quite capture the meaning Pacific people attach to it.

The Fijian term *veitokoni* – mutual support built around dependant relationships – captures the communal nature of Fijian culture. Reciprocity is indicative of families functioning well (New Zealand Ministry of Social Development, 2012). Niueans show reciprocity through *felagomatai* (helping one another), *fekapitigaaki* (having friendly relations) and *fakafeheleaki* (sharing), each vital to maintaining relationships (New Zealand Ministry of Social Development, 2012).

Respect (*fa'aaloaloa* – Sāmoan, *vakarokoroko* – Fijian, *fakaaloaloa* – Tokelau), another commonly held value, is shown through appropriate behaviour and language. Values are so embedded in Pacific cultures; behaviours associated with values are exhibited without explanation. Respectful behaviour helps maintain the *vā/wā*.

Mental wellbeing considers factors such as stress, mental disorder, medication, emotions, attitude and the expression of emotion through behaviour. Physical wellbeing includes sleep, diet, medication, housing and physical environment. The fourth *pou* (pole), other, includes factors such as age, sexuality and gender.

The foundation represents family. Traditional Pacific understandings of family include extended family, village and church community (Taule'ale'asumai, 1997; Meleisea & Schoeffel, 1998). This is evidenced through language. Sāmoans have no word for aunt; when referring to their aunt, children will call their aunt by name or *tinā* (mother). Aunts are given the same respect as mothers and share responsibility of providing love and guidance to nephews and nieces (Ledoux-Taua'aletoa, 2013).

The roof of the *fale* represents culture providing shelter and protection, as Pacific cultures held ways of providing both protection and respect within families. Reflecting on roles within Pacific families, we begin to understand the importance of the *Vā* (relationship) between brothers and sisters. Reflecting on the understanding of *'āiga/kāinga/whānau*/family from a Pacific perspective all women are sisters, whether through shared parents, being a cousin or through village or church community. Therefore, in the traditional context, women and children were highly esteemed and afforded protection. All males belong to *'āiga/kāinga/whānau*/families and are respected and loved through *vā* (relationships).

Traditional Sāmoan *fale* has no walls, the surrounds of the *fale* represents the context that *'āiga/kāinga/whānau*/family are situated. This includes components such as politics at a local and national level, economy and environment. It also includes attitudes towards children and women. Each of these components contribute to individual and collective wellbeing. Wellbeing of children and women can be influenced by the way their roles are perceived by their community.

Efi (2009) reinforces the importance of professionals engaging the wider family and community for sustained positive relationship building, speaking to the essence of understanding Pacific communities and families.

> I am not an individual, I am an integral part of the cosmos. I share divinity with my ancestors, the land, the seas and the skies. I am not an individual, because I share a *tofi* (birth right) with my family, my village and my nation, I belong to my family and my family belongs to me. I belong to my village and my village belongs to me, I belong to my nation and my nation belongs to me, this is the essence of my sense of being.
>
> (Efi, 2009)

When supporting Pacific people, social workers should consider using the *Fonofale* for assessment while developing relationships with the lens of the *Vā*. Pivotal to effective assessment is appropriate engagement. The *vā* (Mila-Schaaf, 2006) is the space in human relationships between individuals or groups that holds respect, determining how interaction and behaviours occur. This sacred space requires conscious effort to maintain (Autagavaia, 2001). Taufe'ulungaki (2004) describes signposts for engagement.

> The core values and practices of Pacific communities were all directed at maintaining and promoting relationships. Thus, the essence of any community is the relationships of its members. It is through these relationships that members come to share experiences and memories, shared roots, shared moral concerns, and shared responsibilities and obligations.
> *(Taufe'ulungaki, 2004, p. 10)*

Engaging through the lens of *vā* in social work with women and children provides opportunity and platform for a strengths-based approach (SBA) (Saleebey, 1997). Strengths that already exist are acknowledged, inclusive of support through *'āiga/kāinga/whānau*/family. SBA encourages sustainable interventions for *'āiga/kāinga/whānau*/family. SBA does not overlook risks, but draws attention to factors such as skills, networks and strengths that minimise risk. Do not assume venerating the collective detracts from the importance of individuals.

> When I say that I am not an individual, I do not mean that my individual happiness is not important. The ideals of the family in the Samoan context is shaped by respect for each person's mental, physical, social and spiritual wellbeing. It is the responsibility of the family, especially the heads of the families, to make sure that each person in the family is happy.
> *(Efi, 2009)*

Social workers should engage with *'āiga/kāinga/whanau*/families as collectives, without detracting from the needs and aspirations of women and children (Ledoux-Taua'aletoa, 2013). Pacific leaders, whether they are leaders within their *'āiga/kāinga/whanau*/families or in the wider community, are being challenged to focus on the needs of *'āiga/kāinga/whanau*/families (Failautusi, 2017). Communities and *'āiga/kāinga/whanau*/families have always had leadership structures that provide guidance and protection (Meleisea & Schoeffel, 1998, Ledoux-Taua'aletoa, 2013). Leadership structures remain in place, albeit adapted to changing contemporary needs. Pacific academics challenge family leaders to measure leadership against the following criterion:

1. Are children fed and healthy?
2. Are you (as a leader) healthy?
3. Are the aged cared for?
4. Do children and women live without fear?

(Failautusi, 2017)

This challenge acknowledges collective responsibility for women and children.

CASE STUDY 11.1: CHILD PROTECTION

This case study is based in an Aotearoa New Zealand statutory child protection context. I am a social work co-worker. A referral is received from school with concerns for a student. The key worker is a Maori/Samoan male. We conduct a home visit with mother (Lisa), father (Tony) and uncle (Bob) present. The child (Eva) is at school. Eva 10-year-old girl of Cook Island descent. Born in Aotearoa/New Zealand, she speaks English and Rarotongan Cook Island. After receiving a referral from Eva's school, initial checks are made of the records held by child protection services in New Zealand. Tony was released from prison after serving a sentence for illegal sexual connection (rape) of his older daughter (Sala). Eva lives with both parents and Bob. The adults speak both English and Rarotongan Cook Island. Sala does not live in the family home. Tony has tried to mend his relationship with Sala, the relationship remains difficult with Sala limiting contact. Tony respects this decision. Lisa is present but only responds to direct questions, answers are brief. Tony and Bob are fully engaged. We need a clearer understanding of the relationships and roles within the house.

- How is Bob related – maternal or paternal uncle?

If Bob is a maternal uncle can we attribute Lisa's level of participation to her brother providing a voice for her?

If he is a paternal uncle (Tony's brother), is Lisa's level of participation due to her feeling powerless?

- What is the wider family involvement?

Tony and Bob have already mentioned that Tony is actively involved with his family.

- What is Bob's role?

Bob could be living in the home to support Lisa and Eva if he is Lisa's brother, or to support Eva and Tony if he is Tony's brother.

- Is this family involved in a church community?
- Is Lisa free to participate?

A decision is made for me to speak separately with Lisa. Things to consider:

- Bob, Tony and Lisa are cooperative and Lisa is given an opportunity to speak with me separately. She will not share more than what she feels safe to share, i.e. she does not "know me".
- Even if Bob is Lisa's brother we can't assume that he's protective of her and Eva.

Lisa engages, talking about the impact of Tony's offending on her self-esteem in her sexual performance and protecting Sala. Lisa spoke about Bob's ongoing support during Tony's incarceration. His protective relationship with both Eva and Sala empowered them to build strong trusting relationships with men. The extended family provide support to Eva, Sala and Lisa and they have a strong church community that provide ongoing support. Prior to Tony returning home, Eva had been sleeping in Lisa's room. Lisa and Eva developed a close relationship. Eva has returned to sleeping in her room. This has resulted in Eva becoming unsettled. In the bigger meeting, Lisa felt that Bob represented her well. Bob had Lisa and Eva's interests at heart. Other things Lisa wanted to contribute had sexual content inappropriate for discussion in front of males.

REFLECTIVE QUESTIONS

1. What are the impacts on Lisa and Eva's wellbeing?
2. Spiritually: How will you gauge spiritual wellbeing?
3. Mentally: Do the women and children live free of fear?
4. Physically: Are the adults healthy? Are the children fed and healthy?

Conclusion

Globally, conventions and strategies are in place to improve the position of women and children. Across the region, tradition and proverbs provide insights to how children and women are esteemed, although colonisation has had significant effect on the position of women and children today. There are positive challenges from within Pacific communities that call on Pacific people to re-evaluate leadership against specific criteria. The criteria promote and enhance the wellbeing of women and children, aligning better with traditions held prior to colonisation. Pacific communities and families have within their traditions values and principles that should be used as a vehicle for successful, sustainable change. Engagement is the key for gathering information that will inform assessments for effectively working with Pacific families and communities.

References

Anae, M. (2016). Teu Le Vā: Samoan relational ethics. *Knowledge Cultures*, 4(3), 117–130.

Autagavaia, M. (2001). Social work with Pacific Island communities. In M. Connolly (Ed.). *New Zealand social work: Contexts and practice* (pp. 72–84). Auckland, New Zealand: Oxford University Press.

Bronfenbrenner, U. (1990). Discovering what families do. In *Rebuilding the nest: A new commitment to the American family*. Milwaukee, WI: Family Service America.

Cumming, G. S. & Allen, C. R. (2017). Protected areas as social-ecological systems: Perspectives from resilience and social-ecological systems theory. *Ecological Applications*, 27(6), 1709–1717. doi:10.1002/eap.1584

Efi, T. A. T. T. T. (2009). Head of State of the Independent State of Samoa: Speech at the New Zealand Families Commission Pasifika Families' Fono, Telstra Clear Pacific events centre, Manukau City, November 3, 2009. Retrieved from www.suawilliamsio.co.nz/?p=643

Endemann-Pulotu, K. (2001). Fonofale Health Research Model. Retrieved from https://religiondocbox.com/Alternative_Religions/70327180-Fonofale-model-of-health-by-fuimaono-karl-pulotu-endemann-as-at-september-2001.html

Failautusi, P. A. (2017, 24 November). Speech presented at Samoan Transnational Fa'amatai Symposium in Auckland University, Auckland.

Helu, F. (1995). Brother/sister and gender relations in ancient and modern Tonga. *Journal de la Société des océanistes*, 100(1), 191–200. DOI: 10.3406/jso.1995.1963

Ledoux-Taua'aletoa, S. M. (2013). *An exploration into the ways in which multi-generational Samoan households contribute to the development of societal and collective values about Aiga/families in contemporary New Zealand/Aotearoa/Niu Sila* (Master's thesis, Unitec, Auckland, New Zealand). Retrieved from http://unitec.researchbank.ac.nz/handle/10652/2316

McMahon, M. O. (1996). *The general method of social work practice: A problem-solving approach* (3rd ed.). Englewood Cliffs, NJ: Prentice Hall.

Meleisea, M. & Schoeffel, P. (1998). Samoan families in New Zealand: The cultural context of change. In V. Adair & R. Dixon (Eds.). *The family in Aotearoa New Zealand*. Auckland, New Zealand: Longman Publishers.

Mila-Schaaf, K. (2006). Va-centred social work possibilities for a Pacific approach to social work practice. *Social Work Review (Tu Mau II)*, 18(1), 8–13.

Ministry of Social Development NZ (2012). *Nga vaka o kaiga tapu: Pasefika proud family violence research plan 2013–2018*. Ministry of Social Development NZ, (October).

Nash, M., Munford, R. & O'Donoghue, K. (Eds.). (2005). *Social work theories in action*. London: Jessica Kingsley Publishers.

New Zealand Ministry of Social Development. (2012). *Nga vaka o kaiga tapu: A Pacific conceptual framework to address family violence in New Zealand*. Auckland, New Zealand: Ministry of Social Development.

Pacific Community & United Nations Human Rights. (2016). *Human rights in the Pacific: A situational analysis*. Noumea: Author.

Papali'i, F. (2017). Samoan Transnational Fa'amatai Symposium. 24 November 2017, Auckland University Keynote Speaker.

Saleebey, D. (1997). The strengths approach to practice. In D. Saleebey (Ed.). *Strengths perspective in social work practice* (2nd ed., pp. 49–57). White Plains, NY: Longman.

Tamasese, K., Peteru, C. and Waldegrave, C. (1997). *Ole Taeoa Afua: The new Morning: A qualitative investigation into Samoan perspectives on mental health and culturally appropriate services*. Wellington, New Zealand: The Family Centre.

Tanjasiri, S.P., Wallace, S.P. and Shibata, K. (1995). Picture imperfect: Hidden problems among Asian Pacific Islander elderly. *The Gerontologist*, 35(6), 753–760. doi.org/10.1093/geront/35.6.753

Taufe'ulungaki, A. (2004). Fonua: Reclaiming Pacific communities in Aotearoa. In *Lotu Moui: Keynote speeches* (pp. 1–6). Auckland, New Zealand: Counties Manukau District Health Board.

Taule'ale'ausumai, F. (1997). The word made flesh: A Samoan theology of pastoral care. In P. Culberston (Ed.). *Counselling issues and South Pacific communities*. Auckland, New Zealand: Snedden & Cervin Publishing Limited.

Thaman, K. H. (2003). Decolonizing Pacific studies: Indigenous perspectives, knowledge, and wisdom in higher education. *The Contemporary Pacific, 15*(1), 1–17. https://doi.org/10.1353/cp.2003.0032

World Health Organisation. (2018). *Adolescent mental health*. Retrieved from www.who.int/mental_health/maternal-child/adolescent/en/

12
AN INTRODUCTION TO SEXUAL AND REPRODUCTIVE HEALTH AND WELLBEING FOR PACIFIC SOCIAL WORK

Michelle Redman-MacLaren and Analosa Veukiso-Ulugia

Key points

1. Be introduced to the definitions of sexual and reproductive health and wellbeing;
2. Learn why sexual and reproductive health and wellbeing are central to holistic social work practice;
3. Explore sexual and reproductive health issues facing Pacific peoples, including cultural, social and religious influences;
4. Learn from a sexual health practitioner from Aotearoa New Zealand who works with Pacific young people;
5. Explore implications for social work practice of policy relating to Pacific sexual and reproductive health and wellbeing;
6. Critically reflect about your own experiences of sexual and reproductive health to ensure safety for the Pacific peoples you work with.

A STORY

Jeanie[1] is a young woman in her late teens who lives in a small timber house roofed with iron. Her village was built by an oil palm plantation company that operates on the outskirts of Popondetta, Oro Province, Papua New Guinea (PNG). This house has two small rooms with a narrow entrance-way tenuously holding the stairs in its meagre arms. There is no kitchen inside – the cooking takes place on an open fire in the makeshift outdoor kitchen, squeezed between Jeanie's house and her neighbour's.

> Jeanie's parents work as field workers in the oil palm plantation, returning at night to the company village. Jeanie has had limited educational opportunities. Jeanie attended school until she was 12 years old, when her parents decided she would be more useful staying at home to carry water, help care for her younger siblings and prepare meals. This freed Jeanie's mother to return to the plantation, bringing in much needed cash. Leaving school at the age of 12 is a common pattern where Jeanie lives. Half the number of girls compared with boys finish high school in PNG.
>
> Jeanie has a boyfriend (that her parents do not know about); while Jeanie knows about *SikAIDS*[2] (HIV and AIDS) and male circumcision, she cannot talk about these things with her boyfriend as she is just a "single girl" and circumcision *em sumting blong olgeta man* (is men's business) (Redman-MacLaren, 2015).

Sexual and reproductive health and wellbeing – An introduction

As social workers, we have the privilege of working alongside individuals, families and their communities across the life span. Each developmental stage presents unique issues for the people we work with. For most, sexual and reproductive health and wellbeing is a central concern from late childhood, through adolescence, middle and into older age. However, as social workers, how well equipped are we to talk about sex with those we work with? How do we approach topics that may be considered taboo?

In this chapter, you will find a range of terms used, including sex, sexuality, sexual health and sexual wellbeing. These terms mean different things to different people. Our understanding of these terms are influenced by our upbringing, families, schools, friends, social technology, and as a result of our work (Bywater & Jones, 2007). Therefore, it is important to establish a shared understanding of what we mean when we talk about sexual and reproductive health and wellbeing.

Sexual and reproductive health and wellbeing

Let's start with wellbeing. Wellbeing, especially for Pacific peoples, is holistic and encompasses emotional, physical, spiritual and psychological aspects of life (Pulotu-Endemann, 2009). Central to the concept of Pacific wellbeing is the importance of relational harmony – symmetry between an individual and their relationships with others (such as family members), and their relationships with the natural and spiritual environment (Percival, et al., 2010; Pulotu-Endemann, 2009).

Sexual wellbeing refers to how we experience our sexual selves and our relationships with others, with Jeanie's story one example of this. A wide range of values, attitudes and behaviours make up sexual wellbeing; it is complex and multifaceted. A useful glossary of key sexual terms and conceptual elements that include sex, sexual health and sexual rights were developed by the Pan American Health Organisation (PAHO) and the World Health Organisation (WHO) (World Health Organisation, 2006). For the purposes of this chapter, we use the WHO definition of sexuality:

> Sexuality is a central aspect of being human throughout life encompasses sex, gender identities and roles, sexual orientation, eroticism, pleasure, intimacy and reproduction. Sexuality is experienced and expressed in thoughts, fantasies, desires, beliefs, attitudes, values, behaviours, practices, roles and relationships. While sexuality can include all of these dimensions, not all of them are always experienced or expressed. Sexuality is influenced by the interaction of biological, psychological, social, economic, political, cultural, legal, historical, religious and spiritual factors.
>
> *(World Health Organisation, 2006)*

Sexuality encompasses a broad spectrum of beliefs, motivations, values and actions. Sexuality includes important behaviours and outcomes, such as pregnancy and sexual infections. While there is a relationship between sexual health and reproductive health, there are also important differences (Browne, 2017). Reproductive health addresses the reproductive processes, functions and systems at all stages of life (WHO, 2018). This includes a focus on the reproductive system: the system or organs which fulfil reproductive functions and processes. In males, this includes but is not limited to penis and testes. For females, it includes the ovaries and uterus. However, sexual health has a broader focus that extends beyond the reproductive system, such as sexual relationships, sexual assault and violence, mental health, sexual orientation and gender identity" (Secretariat of the Pacific Community, 2015).

Why is sexual health important?

Sexual health influences not only the physical, emotional and spiritual wellbeing of individuals, but families and our wider community. When individuals, couples and families experience good sexual health, the social and economic development of communities and countries is also positively impacted (WHO, 2010). However, the experience of good sexual health and wellbeing relies upon being able to make healthy choices. Three interrelated features assist to achieve this outcome (see Table 12.1) (SPC, 2014).

We, as social workers, can positively support these features of good sexual health.

TABLE 12.1 Interrelated features required to experience positive sexual health

1. Individuals and families have appropriate and comprehensive knowledge and information about sexual health and related risks,
2. Access to high-quality health services and commodities and
3. An enabling environment that promotes good sexual health and wellbeing for all without discrimination (Secretariat of the Pacific Community, 2014, p. 13).

Sexual and reproductive health in social work practice

"Social work is not just about problem issues in relation to sexuality, but about positively promoting sexual well-being" (Bywater & Jones, 2007, p. 133). The global definition of social work developed by the International Association of Schools of Social Work (IASSW) General Assembly and the International Federation of Social Workers (IFSW) charges social workers to engage with people and structures to address life challenges and enhance wellbeing (IFSW, 2014). An important component captured in the global definition is that our practice is to be underpinned by core theories, including indigenous knowledges. In addition, the amplified definition of social work developed specifically for the Asia Pacific region (APASWE, 2016) highlights five key areas unique to Asia Pacific. These areas include the importance of faith, spirituality and religion in people's lives and the need to respect varying belief systems. In addition, social workers in Asia Pacific are tasked to engage in critical and research-based practice, and to affirm indigenous and local knowledges (APASWE, 2016).

Social workers have the potential to contribute to each of the interrelated features necessary to experience positive sexual health (see Table 12.1). We can: a) ensure our clients have appropriate and comprehensive information about sexual health and related risks; b) advocate for the provision of high-quality health services; and c) become actively involved in developing enabling environments that encourage good sexual health and wellbeing.

Social workers are not usually trained to be sex therapists or psychosexual counsellors and can find this field challenging (Christopher, 1980). However, if a social worker discovers there is a sexual or reproductive health problem, they can work with the person/s to identify strategies to address these issues. If both agree, a referral may be made to another service or agency. If there is a reluctance to seek help, we as social workers can continue to work alongside that person/s, fully aware of our professional boundaries.

This section has highlighted sexual health concepts and the interface with social work practice. The following task invites you to reflect on these ideas by considering your understanding of terms used in sexual and reproductive health.

> **REFLECTION**
>
> Reflect upon your understanding of the following sexual terms. Who and what do you think have influenced your understanding?
>
> **Sexual terms**
>
> | | | |
> |---|---|---|
> | Sex | Heterosexual | Homophobia |
> | Sexuality | Bisexual | Heterosexism |
> | Sexual orientation | Transgender | Homosexual |
> | Gender | Gay | Lesbian |
> | Fa'afafine | Fakaleiti | Mahu Wahine |
> | Mahu Vahine | Rae Rae | Vaka sa lewa lewa |
> | Pinapinaaine | Fafafine | Akava'ine |
> | Girly Girly | | |
>
> Should we as social workers discuss family planning methods and contraceptive counselling with our clients? Do you believe the people we work with should discuss family planning and contraceptive methods with their families?
>
> *(Adapted from Bywater & Jones, 2007, p. 2)*

Pacific sexual and reproductive health and wellbeing

Sexual and reproductive health and wellbeing (SRH&W) in the Pacific is influenced by a diverse range of social, cultural and spiritual factors, as diverse as the islands that lay in the vast Pacific Ocean. This means the SRH&W needs of Pacific Islander women, men, young people and children are extremely diverse. As social workers, we are adept at assessing individual and family needs as they are expressed within communities and systems. Actions to improve sexual health, for example, can take place within a range of settings, including reproductive health programmes, through primary health care or through other settings including education, social welfare and youth programmes (WHO, 2010). When addressing complex challenges as social workers, a multi-sectoral approach works best. As social workers enacting a systems response, we require skills that include sensitivity to social, cultural and spiritual influences on SRH&W, as evidenced in Jeanie's story.

What are the SRH&W issues in the Pacific?

In the Pacific region, sexual issues include high rates of sexually transmitted infections (STIs), increasing numbers of people living with Human

Immunodeficiency Virus (HIV), gender-based violence and sexual assault, high rates of adolescent pregnancy and low levels of use of contraceptives (SPC, 2014). Addressing SRH&W of Pacific peoples is an urgent priority.

In Pacific cultures that do not always promote open discussion about sexual health (Queensland Health, 2011; Veukiso-Ulugia, 2016), there is opportunity to address sexual health issues through the reproductive health agenda. This approach is encouraged by the World Health Organisation (2010), but there is a risk that a focus on the "reproductive" will exclude other important sexual health issues (Browne, 2017). This is particularly important for people for whom reproductive health may not be the highest priority (for example, members of the rainbow [LGBTQ+] community).

Cultural and spiritual beliefs and practices about sex and reproduction

When reflecting on the similarities and differences between Pacific and Maori communities, a Maori student asked me (AVU), "when did it become shameful to talk about sex in Pacific communities? Was it missionaries and Christianity?" I could have provided a range of answers. We know that despite the diversity of cultural and religious expressions across the Pacific, there are few Pacific cultures that enable free expression of sexuality and the fulfilment of sexual and reproductive health and rights (SPC, 2014, p. 54). Pre-eminent Samoan leader Tui Atua Tupua Tamasese has written extensively on Samoan culture, and specifically about sexuality and sexual behaviour. His insights into traditional sexual values and practices outline that in pre-missionary times, Samoans embraced sexuality, masculinity and femininity (Suaalii-Sauni et al., 2014).

The predominant norms of traditional patriarchal cultures, embedded within contemporary religious practices (most commonly Christianity), contribute to shaping and constraining access to sexual and reproductive health services. Patriarchal practices such as bride price and arranged marriage (for example, in Melanesia) often have advantages for tribes or clans, but can be a precursor to violence against individual women and girls (Shih et al., 2017). Christianity in the Pacific often promotes conservative sexual values espoused by religious communities, talking about sex can elicit shame and access to sexual and reproductive health knowledge and services can be limited (Veukiso-Ulugia, 2016). It is important to consider both the advantages and disadvantages of these ubiquitous and evolving social, cultural and religious systems when working with people from Pacific islands.

> People have sex for a whole range of reasons. Reproduction is one of these reasons but there are many others, including pleasure or to earn an income. In some cases, people are forced to have sex against their will.
>
> *(SPC, 2014, p. 13)*

We know that sexual violence occurs in all countries, including Pacific island countries and territories (Cox, 2010). Evidence shows us that sexual violence often forms a part of women's experience of abuse. In a national survey in Solomon

Islands, 37% of women reported having been sexually abused before the age of 15 (Secretariat of the Pacific Community, 2009). In addition to the psychological distress and social shame that comes from experiencing sexual violence, this violence is linked to other issues, such as sexual and reproductive health rights such as access to safe abortion. Abortion is another taboo subject in many Pacific communities (Vallely et al., 2015). As social workers, we must consider how best to support individuals, their families and communities in these challenging contexts.

As uncomfortable as it might be for some of us, the reality is that many Pacific girls and women, men who have sex with men and transgender women use sex as a commodity. Sex is exchanged for money or goods, often in environments where there is very little employment or social support and is often precipitated by family dislocation, grief, family breakdown, marital separation and/or widowhood (Kelly-Hanku et al, 2018). Selling or exchanging sex can increase the risk of violence, especially against women and girls, as they are viewed as "transgressive" and thus less respected (Kelly-Hanku et al., 2016).

> **REFLECTION**
>
> Across the Pacific, large families are the norm. This norm creates an important social safety net, where everyone is responsible for looking out for each other. However, this cultural norm also brings cultural expectations about sexual relations, marriage and the importance of having children.
>
> How might the cultural expectation for women to have many children affect the realisation of their sexual and reproductive health and rights?

"Don't make it awkward": An interview with Ruth Uo, Team Leader – Youth Fale at Village Collective

She [young person] said, "and so I went to this party and this guy, you know, he got up, getting drunk, and I went with my cousin to this party, I got drunk and then I got with this guy". But the way that she was expressing it to me was a way, she felt like, you could tell she was uncomfortable with it, but she was drunk, she didn't give consent. So she felt really gross afterwards, she [young person] just felt really uneasy about the whole thing, and the thing was, that she said to me that he [this guy] has been asking her if they could do it again. And so she was thinking about it. I asked "Do you feel safe?", she said "I kind of don't".

And so when we think about safety, those are things that are key, as a facilitator, as a person who hears that, we have to actually step in and try to do something, because we're seeing these responses [from young people] to these kind of situations.

(Uo, 2018)

The Village Collective (VC) is a Pacific-centric charitable organisation that works with Pacific youth and families in Auckland, New Zealand. Operating since 1997, the VC team comprised of Pacific sexual health educators, equip Pacific youth, families and communities with the relevant knowledge and resources to achieve good sexual health. In working with hundreds of school students, including Pacific, Ms Uo identified the complexity and sensitivity surrounding sex and wellbeing. Her advice for social workers:

- Be knowledgeable and comfortable in where you yourself stand in relation to sexual health
- Take the time to build relationships and create a safe environment with those you are working with (rather than rushing into providing answers)
- Listen
- Ensure open communication and safety procedures are in place with key professionals (such as social workers, guidance and support staff)
- Get support – from your team – and ensure regular supervision
- Be prepared for the unexpected and the uncomfortable (as evident in the following comment)

> I have learnt not to judge a person by their outward behaviour or manner. There have been occasions when young people in the session do not appear to be engaged or interested in what we are sharing. However, I've had the experience of these same young people in later sessions approaching me to ask questions, and later share they have experienced abuse and not sure if they should be feeling the way they do. I've learnt never to make these assumptions, as they may be processing some very deep traumatic events.
>
> (Uo, 2018)

Consistent with the African proverb, "it takes a village to raise a child", VC's three service fales (houses) Youth, Rainbow and Community metaphorically represent the village that is needed to help communities experience positive sexual health. The Youth fale team provide interactive workshops with students in primary, intermediate, high schools, alternative education and training. The Rainbow fale provides services to those who identify as lesbian, gay, bisexual, transgender, queer, intersex, asexual, fakaleiti, vakasalewalewa, fakafifine, akavaine, drodolagi and mahu. The Community fale collaborates with local communities and external agencies to support their work.

The VC team are culturally diverse, certified and have undertaken graduate training in public health and sexual health. Skilled facilitators, they assist individuals and communities to navigate through complex social, emotional, psychological and cultural issues that arise. VC have developed tailored Pacific resources, including performance pieces such as "Talanoa: Full disclosure without concealment", that highlights the taboo nature of sex, sexuality and relationships drawing on stories from Pacific peoples.

Social work and social policy: the roles we can play to improve SRH&W

> Sexual health requires a positive and respectful approach to sexuality and sexual relationships, as well as the possibility of having pleasurable and safe sexual experiences, free of coercion, discrimination and violence. For sexual health to be attained and maintained, the sexual rights of all persons must be respected, protected and fulfilled.
>
> *(World Health Organisation, 2006, p. 1)*

This statement reflects what is needed to achieve good sexual health. However, how can we as social workers ensure sexual rights are realised, given SRH&W is influenced by an extensive range of factors, including socio-economic status, access to health and education services, gender inequality, and national and international development priorities? (SPC, 2015). While many social workers work largely in micro and meso-system settings, macro-level factors, such as government policies, have a significant impact on SRH&W.

Government policies signal how each country will meet the health and wellbeing needs of its citizens. This is expressed in the kinds of services that are funded, how they are delivered and who can access these services (Maidment & Beddoe, 2009). From a practice perspective, social workers are expected to implement policy in diverse settings including local communities and government agencies, regional and global forums. Our everyday work gives us understanding of how policy impacts clients and communities. We are in a powerful position to advocate for policies and practices that support SRH&W. As advocates we can draw on and respond to the various opportunities available at global, regional and national settings (as highlighted in Table 12.2).

As "agents of change" charged with addressing social injustice, we social workers recognise that policies can either promote wellbeing or unintentionally increase the risk of harm. We now explore how our personal experiences need to be critically reflected upon to ensure we cause no harm to those we with whom we work.

REFLECTION

What are the social policies and/or strategies that refer to SRH&W in your country?

How are Pacific peoples affected by the policy? Is the policy adequately resourced?

How do these policies influence your social work practice?

What are the ways that we as social workers can advocate for and influence positive SRH&W policies?

Identify how you, as a social worker working with Pacific peoples, could influence SRH&W policy practice. Consider how you could contribute to: professional social work associations; advocacy groups; peer support, e.g. Youth Champs, Fiji; Pacific-focused advisory groups; and/or research.

TABLE 12.2 Examples of international, regional and national policy organisations

Setting	Organisation
International	**United Nations** The United Nations (UN) is an intergovernmental organisation that is comprised of 193 member states tasked with promoting international cooperation and order. Examples of declarations and goals with a SRH&W focus include the Universal Declaration of Human Rights and Sustainable Development Goals (SDGs) (United Nations, 2015). **World Association for Sexual Health (WAS)** Established in 1978, the World Association for Sexual Health (WAS) is a global organisation that focuses on sexual health and rights. The Declaration of Sexual Rights, developed by WAS, is an important resource that can aid our understanding of SRH&W (WAS, 2014).
Regional	**World Health Organisation – Western Pacific Region** Within World Health Organization (WHO), responsible for directing and coordinating international health efforts, member states are grouped into six regions. The Western Pacific Region comprises 26 member states that includes Pacific island countries and territories, Aotearoa New Zealand and Australia. The WHO provide routine surveillance of health issues within each of the regions (WHO WPR, 2018). **Pacific Community** The Secretariat of the Pacific Community (SPC) is a regional development organisation established in 1947. SPC is governed by 26 countries, including all 22 Pacific Island countries and territories. SPC has released a number of regional documents related to Pacific sexual health (SPC, 2014).
National (Individual countries)	Most countries have their own policies and strategies to inform responses to SRH&W. For example, in Aotearoa New Zealand, the Sexual and Reproductive Health Strategy (2001) highlights how the government plans to achieve positive and improved sexual and reproductive health for all New Zealanders (Ministry of Health, 2001).

You, the social worker: Critical reflection for purposeful practice in a sensitive field

Social workers will have varying degrees of comfort in discussing sex with their clients. The clients themselves will be sensitive to any discomfort on the part of the social worker and this may inhibit them from revealing the true nature of their difficulties … Thus the social worker should first of all try to make himself (sic) comfortable talking about sex. This of course, is made easier by experience. Practice, practice, practice talking, asking about sex.

(Christopher, 1980, p. 64)

Working in the sexual and reproductive health field is a great privilege, but can also be confronting on many levels. Our personal values, religious beliefs, family history, professional and personal linkages all contribute to what we bring to this aspect of social work practice. We almost certainly will come into contact with beliefs and practices not consistent with our own. Human sexuality is a most intimate and important part of life, and yet, as we have discussed throughout this chapter, it can be shrouded in shame, secrecy and sometimes violence and pain.

As we bring ourselves as social workers to this space, we need to consider how our own beliefs and experiences might impact the way we respond to people experiencing sexual and reproductive health issues, and how we might promote wellbeing for the individuals and communities that we work with. Bywater and Jones remind us as social workers that we "need to be comfortable about your own sexuality in order to be open and sensitive to the sexual issues of other people" (2007, p. 131).

Below is a short exercise in critical reflection, an important social work practice that unearths, examines and changes very deeply held or fundamental assumptions that leads to a change in these assumptions (Fook, 2005).

> **REFLECTION**
>
> Take 10 minutes to write down how sexuality was presented when you were growing up. Did your family talk with you about sex? Were sexual practices viewed as taboo or too shameful to talk about? Have these attitudes changed? Have your attitudes changed? How might your own beliefs and practices about sex influence who you work with and how you work with them?

The preparedness to discuss difficult and sensitive subjects is a professional strength of social workers (Bywaters & Ungar, 2010), but requires we start with critically reflecting upon ourselves, and our own practice. The short poem below describes the transformation that can occur when we stop and critically reflect upon our practice.

> Critical reflection
> You hunt me
> down, and up
> change my path
> challenge my base
> invite a new road
> block an old
> It is time to acknowledge
> I had it wrong
> I am new

Because of you
Critical
Reflection.

Conclusion

Sexual and reproductive health is a continual and critical challenge globally, with peoples of the Pacific experiencing these challenges in a culturally constructed way. As Jeanie's story shows us, limited educational opportunities, cultural and religious norms that privilege patriarchy and limited access to suitable sexual and reproductive health services can impact the wellbeing of those we work with. Social work is uniquely positioned to provide non-judgemental space for the Pacific people we work to navigate this challenging, but rewarding, aspect of health and wellbeing across the lifespan.

In this chapter, you have:

- Learned the definitions of sexual and reproductive health and wellbeing, specifically as they relate to Pacific peoples
- Been introduced to SRH&W issues facing Pacific peoples, including cultural, social and religious influences
- Learned how sexual and reproductive health is pivotal to social work practice
- Read how a Samoan practitioner works with Pacific young people in Aotearoa New Zealand
- Considered social work practice and policy responses to sexual and reproductive health issues in the Pacific
- Been reminded of the importance of critical reflection to safe social work practice in sexual and reproductive health

Notes

1 Jeanie is not a real person, but the facts in this story are.
2 HIV and/or AIDS.

References

APASWE. (2016). *APASW Asia Pacific Association for Social Work Education – Joint Amplification of the Global Definition on Social Work Profession in Asia and Pacific*. Retrieved from www.apaswe.com/index.php/news-event/159-check-it-out-apaswe-no-12-2015-2017

Browne, K. C. (2017). The S in SRH: Sexual health and well-being. *Pacific Journal of Reproductive Health, 1*(5), 240–244.

Bywater, J. & Jones, R. (2007). *Sexuality and social work*. Exeter, United Kingdom: Learning Matters Ltd.

Bywaters, P. & Ungar, M. (2010). Health and well-being. In I. Shaw, K. Briar-Lawson, J. Orme, & R. Ruckdeschel (Eds.), *The SAGE handbook of social work research* (pp. 392–405). London: Sage.

Christopher, E. (1980). *Sexuality and birth control in social and community work*. London: Temple Smith.

Cox, E. (2010). *Ending violence against women and girls: Literature review and annotated bibliography*. Suva, Fiji: UNIFEM, Pacific.
Fook, J. (2005). Reflective practice and critical reflection. In *Handbook for practice learning in social work and social care* (pp. 440–454). J. Lishman (Editor). London: Jessica Kingsley Publishers.
IFSW (International Federation of Social Work) (2014). Global definition of the social work. IFSW general meeting and the IASSW general assembly, July 2014. Retrieved from www.ifsw.org/what-is-social-work/global-definition-of-social-work/
Kelly-Hanku, A., Aeno, H., Wilson, L., Eves, R., Mek, A., Nake Trumb, R., ... Vallely, A. (2016). Transgressive women don't deserve protection: Young men's narratives of sexual violence against women in rural Papua New Guinea. *Culture, Health and Sexuality, 18*(11), 1207–1220.
Kelly-Hanku, A., Amos-Kuma, A., Badman, S. G., Weikum, D., Boli Neo, R., Hou, P., ... Hakim, A. (2017). *Kauntim mi tu – Port Moresby: Key findings from the Key Population Integrated Bio-Behavioural Survey, Port Moresby, Papua New Guinea*. Papua New Guinea Institute of Medical Research and Kirby Institute, UNSW Sydney: Goroka, Papua New Guinea.
Kelly-Hanku, A., Willie, B., Weikum, D.,A., Boli Neo, R., Kupul, M., Coy, K., Hou, P., Aeno. H., Ase, S., Gabuzzi, J., Nembari, J., Narakobi, R., Amos-Kuma, A., Gare, J., Dala, N., Wapling, J., Toliman, P., John, L., Nosi, S., Worth, H., Whiley, D., Tabrizi, S.N, Kaldor, J.M., Vallely, A.J, Badman, S.G. and Hakim, A. (2018). Kauntim mi tu: Multi-site summary report from the key population integrated bio-behavioural survey, Papua New Guinea. Goroka, Papua New Guinea: Papua New Guinea Institute of Medical Research and Kirby Institute, UNSW Sydney.
Maidment, J. & Beddoe, E. (2009). *Mapping knowledge for social work practice. Critical intersections*. South Melbourne, Australia: Cengage Learning.
Ministry of Health. (2001). *Sexual and reproductive health strategy: Phase one*. Wellington, New Zealand: Ministry of Health.
Percival, T., Robati-Mani, R., Powell, E., Kingi, P., Peteru, M. C., Hope, L.-T., ... Rankine, J. (2010). *Pacific pathways to the prevention of sexual violence: Full report*. Auckland, New Zealand: Pacific Health, School of Population Health, University of Auckland.
Pulotu-Endemann, F. K. (2009). *Fonofale model of health*. Retrieved from www.hauora.co.nz/resources/Fonofalemodelexplanation.pdf
Queensland Health. (2011). *Queensland Health response to Pacific Islander and Māori health needs assessment*. Retrieved from www.health.qld.gov.au/__data/assets/pdf_file/0037/385867/qh-response-data.pdf
Redman-MacLaren, M. (2015). *The implications of male circumcision practices for women in Papua New Guinea, including for HIV prevention* (pp. 1–341). Doctor of Philosophy, James Cook University. Retrieved from https://researchonline.jcu.edu.au/42315/
Secretariat of the Pacific Community (2009). *Solomon Islands Family Health and Safety Study: A study on violence against women and children*. Noumea, Secretariat of the Pacific Community. Retrieved from www.spc.int/hdp/index2.php?option=com_docman&task=doc_view&gid=49&
Secretariat of the Pacific Community. (2014). *Pacific sexual health and well being shared agenda 2015–2019*. Retrieved from www.spc.int/hiv/index.php?option=com_docman&task=cat_view&gid=182&Itemid=148
Secretariat of the Pacific Community. (2015). *Awareness. Analysis. Action: Sexual and reproductive health and rights in the Pacific*. Retrieved from http://rrrt.spc.int/publications-media/publications/item/619-awareness-analysis-action-sexual-reproductive-health-and-rights-in-the-pacific

Shih, P., Worth, H., Travaglia, J. & Kelly-Hanku, A. (2017). "Good culture, bad culture": Polygyny, cultural change and structural drivers of HIV in Papua New Guinea. *Culture, Health & Sexuality, 19*(9), 1024–1037. doi:10.1080/13691058.2017.1287957

Suaalii-Sauni, T. M., Wendt, M. A., Fuamatu, N., Va'ai, U. L., Whaitiri, R. & Filipo, S. L. (2014). *Whispers and vanities: Samoan indigenous knowledge and religion*, Wellington, Aotearoa New Zealand: Huia Publishers.

United Nations. (2015). *Sustainable development goals – 17 global goals to transform our world.* Retrieved from www.un.org/sustainabledevelopment/sustainable-development-goals/

Uo, R. (2018, April 12). Personal interview.

Vallely, L. M., Homiehombo, P., Kelly-Hanku, A. & Whittaker, A. (2015). Unsafe abortion requiring hospital admission in the Eastern Highlands of Papua New Guinea – A descriptive study of women's and health care workers' experiences. *Reproductive Health, 12*(22), 1–11.

Veukiso-Ulugia, A. (2016). Good Samoan kids – Fact or fable? Sexual health behaviour of Samoan youth in Aotearoa New Zealand. *New Zealand Sociology, 31*(2), 74–95.

World Association for Sexual Health. (2014). *World Association for Sexual Health – Declaration of Sexual Rights.* Retrieved from www.worldsexology.org/wp-content/uploads/2013/08/declaration_of_sexual_rights_sep03_2014.pdf

World Health Organization (2006). *Sexual and reproductive health – Defining sexual health.* Retrieved from www.who.int/reproductivehealth/topics/sexual_health/sh_definitions/en/

World Health Organization. (2018). *Health topics: Reproductive health.* www.who.int/topics/reproductive_health/en/

World Health Organization Department of Reproductive Health and Research. (2010). *Developing sexual health programmes: A framework for action.* Retrieved from www.who.int/reproductivehealth/publications/sexual_health/rhr_hrp_10_22/en/

World Health Organisation – Western Pacific Region. (2018). *Division of Pacific Technical Support*, Retrieved from www.wpro.who.int/southpacific/en/

13

GETTING ON THE K.A.D.

The impacts of kava, alcohol and other drug consumption across Pacific communities

Moses Ma'alo Faleolo and Jioji Ravulo

Key points

- It is important to have a broader view as to why people consume substances, which includes understanding the socio-cultural context.
- Some of the prevalent substances consumed by Pacific communities include alcohol, tobacco, betel nut and kava, with the later substance tied to traditional and ceremonial purposes.
- Creating and implementing policies and practices that are underpinned by harm minimisation strategies alongside cultural perspectives can assist in decreasing problematic consumption.

Substance use and Pacific social work

The use of substances across the Pacific has a strong historical context from natural and traditional approaches in concert with cultural views connecting with each other and reiterating the importance of peers and community. Various ceremonies have been supported by the use of substances that have then assisted in celebrating important and mementos occasions, to the observance of life through the farewelling of a loved one. Treaties and the creation of binding agreements are also founded through the exchange and use of plants and their products to further forge future connections and allies. However, it is through the excessive and harmful use of certain substances that may create tensions on the utility and usefulness of such practices. This chapter will explore the need to understand the various contexts in which alcohol and other drugs, including traditional substances like kava, are used in and across Pacific communities. The varying roles that these substances play in Pacific cultures and modern society are unpacked, with a view to further incorporate a more inclusive and balanced understanding, especially when it comes to developing meaningful approaches to include or desist from problematic consumption within a social work lens.

In general, Pacific social work practice, policy and research should include these varying perspectives, and navigate and support the individual, family and collective views in which substances are used. In saying this, common social work and public health approaches in this field of practice generally lends itself to prompting an individualistic understanding as to why people may consume in a negative manner, but in a Pacific context, this should be broadened to not just include the socio-economic view on health and wellbeing, but also the socio-cultural perspective on how traditional culture intersects with alcohol and other drugs.

Social work theories in consideration and context

From an intervention perspective, if an individual is experiencing problems with alcohol and other drug usage, then a crisis/task-centred approach may be utilised to support the need to further unpack the impact of such usage in wellbeing. This may be further underpinned by the narrative approach, where the person is given the scope to understand the circumstances that has led to excessive and problematic patterns of substance use, and how this then shapes their own responsibility to such behaviour. This can also be paired with behavioural theory via other forms of talking therapies through the practice of cognitive behaviour therapy (CBT) where an individual or family further discussed their thoughts (cognitions), feelings (emotions) and behaviours (actions) that may lead to alcohol and/or other drug usage, and the possible solutions that may be developed to counteract these responses. Motivational interviewing can also be helpful in the context of promoting positive recovery away from excessive usage, as it potentially unlocks underlying reasons for usage, and then again refocuses on the need to find and source solutions moving forward.

Bringing this into a Pacific context, apart from placing a collective view on the narratives being explored by the individual on the influence of peers and family on usage, it is also important to highlight a shared and communal response. Alcohol and other drug usage have generally been a polarised topic as either a criminal, moral or health issue, with public health messages sharing the same level of mixed conviction. However, it is just as important to understand the role substances play in the Pacific cultural context first, before relegating the approach as one view alone. It is also of importance that interventions are implemented in this way of thinking too; where individuals, families and communities create a shared and meaningful response to using substances and managing the possible adverse effects this has across society.

Prevalent substances across Pacific communities

The following section overviews the various substances that are prevalent across the Pacific region, and most commonly used by Pacific communities in their country of origins, or the diaspora globally. Certain trends have been researched, acknowledging the intersecting role of traditional cultural practice as a means to consume substances as part of a collective context. Rather than participating in substance usage within an individual context alone, there are ongoing parallels with the social use of substances enabling many Pacific people to consume and use as part of the communal connection to self and others (Mission Australia & Ravulo, 2009).

Alcohol

With the formal introduction of alcohol by colonisation in the Pacific, alcohol has become successively more available over time. Certain restrictions have been applied during the evolving use of alcohol in Pacific societies, including specific restrictions placed in village life by Chiefs (Nosa et al., 2018) to the more modern use of alcohol in settings like bars, pubs and clubs. General availability and the shifting acceptance of using alcohol has also changed the way in which Pacific communities have consumed; with some using alcohol instead of traditional substances like kava or home brew. Alcohol has then also become a gateway to enhance social interactions amongst individuals, but once again consumed in the context of a community gathering where people will drink to be included, rather than withdraw.

Marijuana

The use of marijuana has varied across Pacific Island nations and territories, with accessibility to such crops evident in various locations. With the tropical climate in these areas being more suitable for growing such plants, marijuana usage has been used in both an experimental and excessive manner across the Islands. Despite being illegal, marijuana has been incorporated in various sub-cultures in the Pacific including activities related to genres of music; and along with tobacco may act as a gateway to the negative usage of other illicit substances if available (Glover et al., 2011).

Betel nut

Grown and available also in various parts of the Pacific, Betel nut is the seed of the fruit of the areca palm tree. Betel nut is generally consumed orally by chewing the substance wrapped up in the betel leaf, and often accompanied by lime and other flavours to enhance the taste. People will generally feel a slight sense of euphoria or buzz, with usage attached to social or cultural practices (Quinn et al., 2017). Various Pacific Islands have used this substance in various ways, including Federated States of Micronesia, Vanuatu and the Solomon Islands.

Tobacco

Readily available like alcohol, tobacco through products like cigarettes have become widely available in Oceania, with such products generally being cheaper in the Pacific Islands than in Australia and New Zealand. Generally imported from overseas, some tobacco companies have set up factories in the region, including Fiji. The use of e-cigarettes or vaping are a growing trend globally, and has also had a popular uptake in the Pacific region (Kerr, 2018).

Kava

Kava is a beverage that is consumed both socially and traditionally in many Pacific Island nations across Oceania. Many Pacific people understand and utilise the unique properties of kava for use in traditional healing and in the maintenance of cultural identity and practices (Lindstrom, 2009). In Fiji, Sevusevu (kava presentation ritual) is a component of all rituals relating to; culture, all living things, ancestral links and varying forms of spirituality (Shaver & Sosis, 2014). In Sāmoa, an 'Ava (kava) ceremony will take place for all formal occasions including the bestowal of a chief's title, entertaining revered guests and for all significant gatherings. In Tonga, kava ceremonies are seen as a reinforcer of cultural values and ideology. According to Her Royal Highness Princess Salote Mafile'o Pilolevu Tuita, when speaking of the Royal kava ceremony, she relays that kava has special significance to Tongans because it symbolises allegiance, solidarity, the commitment of Tongans to their country, echoes and imparts culture and reasserts loyalty to each other and also to the King (Smith, 2011). Polynesian scholar Futa Helu conveys that customary rituals such as kava ceremonies are not only about learning within one's cultural sphere, but also invites others to learn about that particular society. Helu deems kava ceremonies as the centrepiece of Tongan culture and rituals (Smith, 2011).

The use of kava has proven to be beneficial for treatment in areas such as anxiety, stress-related disorders and stress-induced insomnia with clinical trials suggesting kava is effective for treating anxiety (Cassileth, 2011). Fehoko (2015) highlights the socio-cultural benefits of kava club sessions or "cultural classrooms" in New Zealand where teaching and reinforcing and maintaining the Tongan culture and language is played out in the form of debates, songs and music for both Pacific Island and New Zealand-born males. These findings all suggest that the need for further study into the implementation of kava as an intervention may be useful. However, not all studies and experiences show beneficial effects with little or no side effects.

In New Zealand, in a survey on 12 Tongan men, Nosa and Ofanoa (2009) found that binge-drinking kava was commonplace and entailed drinking from late at night to the early hours of the morning, having a detrimental effect on the family. Nosa and Ofanoa (2009) add that their kava-using participants acknowledged that after consuming kava they felt lethargic and needed a whole day to recover from the effects of kava. Some participants in their study indicated that this negative effect manifested in the form of domestic conflict, resulting in family court action and broken homes (Nosa & Ofanoa, 2009).

Problems with substance misuse

Studies of Pacific Islanders born abroad, including New Zealand, Australia and the USA, provide some insights into the impact of changing economic circumstances and mobility. Existing research highlights unique context-driven risk and protective factors beneficial for illustrating uniquely Pacific issues. The study by Schmich and Power (2010) flagged community policing programmes, peace keeping, industry-specific migrant labour and the return of "troubled" youth to the care of extended families in the Islands as issues of concern relevant to alcohol and other drug (AOD) use. Faleolo's (2016) study of Sāmoan bloods youth gang members in New Zealand found cases of involuntary return migration was partly due to parents being concerned over their teenage children's abuse of alcohol and drugs. He also found that extended families in Sāmoa were ill equipped in managing these troubled youth sent to them from New Zealand. Significantly, Kahn and Fua (1995) identified that amongst Pacific people living in Australia, parental disciplinary methods impacted heavily upon the likelihood of youth involvement in problematic behaviours, particularly substance use.

Schmich and Power (2010) also identified alcohol – licit and illicit (homebrew) – and cannabis as the substances of greatest concern. These findings are based on youth risk behaviour surveys in Vanuatu, Tonga and Micronesia; media reports; and key informant questionnaires and interviews. The importation of alcohol and tobacco continues to be a problem for many Pacific Islands states and territories. Furthermore, heavy alcohol use continues to be a problem, and a number of alcohol-related problems such as drinking and driving, physical violence, mental health and heavy binge drinking continue to be major issues in the region (Devaney et al., 2006; Secretariat of the Pacific Community, 2005).

CASE STUDY 13.1: KAVA CONSUMPTION

In New Zealand, there is very little quantitative evidence relating to the adverse effects of kava consumption. A case study at Middlemore Hospital, New Zealand, provides some insight into the adverse effects of kava usage.

Dr Giles Chanwai reported on the admission of a 34-year-old Tongan male (Patient X) to the Emergency Department at Middlemore Hospital (Chanwai, 2000). Patient X had moved to New Zealand about a month prior and after a night of binge drinking kava, was found by family members very unwell and complaining of sore eyes, headache, generalised muscle weakness, disorientation, hallucinating and abdominal pain. Upon examination he was disorientated around time and place but spoke clearly and followed commands albeit slowly. He was unable to walk or stand, exhibited scaly skin on hands and feet, had little amount of fat over moderate muscle mass, had bloodshot eyes and experienced muscle weakness in the limbs. Prior to Patient X's admission, he reported to being generally well but also communicated to staff that he drank up to 40 bowls of kava per day over the past 14 years. Diagnosis was "kava intoxication on a background of chronic kava consumption" and treated with plasmalyte intravenously and a single dose of thiamine, upon which he improved (Chanwai, 2000).

The reaction Patient X had to excessive kava consumption may be a result of what is termed Pavlovian conditioning and drug tolerance. Although kava is considered a non-narcotic, the consumer does experience a physiological response. Siegel's studies found that conditioned responses were stimulated in situations where drug-associated cues were present and consequently the effect of the drug lessened. This enables drug users to increase the amount of drug dosage with little effect in the same situation or context. However, when the situation, context or environment is altered, drug-associated cues will no longer be present and may lead to an overdose, as the body is not prepared for the drug dosage (Siegel, 2001). So in the case of Patient X being admitted to Middlemore Hospital with kava intoxication, a possible reason for this may be that he was used to consuming a large amount of kava over a prolonged period of time in his native Tonga. Except when Patient X relocated to New Zealand, the context in which he consumed kava altered.

Another aspect may be in relation to acculturation. Acculturation entails people of varying cultures and backgrounds coming together and altering their life long behaviour and culture, culminating in a new society. According to Sam and Berry (2006), early ideology surrounding acculturation considered assimilation to be the ideal form of acculturation as migrants would be better to embrace the new culture and leave behind their own to eliminate acculturative stress. However, such contemporary research suggests that preserving one's heritage and belief systems leads to better adaptation (Sam and Berry, 2010). A four-fold approach to acculturation portrays the way in which an immigrant may respond to their new cultural environment. The four areas are defined as: assimilation – the individual embraces the new culture and belief systems over their own culture; separation – the individual holds firmly to their culture of origin; integration – the individual finds balance between both original and new culture, developing biculturalism; and marginalisation – the individual rejects both cultures for various reasons.

Moving to a new country may be extremely stressful especially when there are language barriers to overcome. Ward (2001) suggests that three specific psychological areas are affected during the migration process including: stress and coping; cultural learning; and social identification. Immigrants face psychological and behavioural changes, which may include adjusting to a new language, clothing differences and dietary variances that may be experienced as minor behavioural changes or at the extreme, problematic adjustment causing "acculturative stress".

> Acculturative stress may manifest in a variety of ways including depression, angst and insecurity (Sam & Berry, 2006). It is possible that due to the acculturation process that Patient X was undergoing, he may have been experiencing acculturative stress with a heightened biological response to the kava consumed despite kava consumption having little effect prior to migration.

Developing and implementing effective AOD policy and practice

What might a harm reduction policy related to kava consumption in the Pacific Islands nations actually look like? What about for alcohol and drug consumption? Will it be the same in the host countries that Pacific Island migrants have resettled in? For alcohol and other drug consumption, harm minimisation is an overarching strategy that aims to prevent and reduce the myriad of social costs associated with usage. It has often been said that the goal of drug policy should be to reduce or minimise the harm associated with drug use rather than reduce or minimise drug use itself. Harm minimisation comprises three major strategies: 1) harm reduction, 2) supply reduction and 3) demand reduction (Australian Government Department of Health, 2004). The concept of harm minimisation appears relatively new for policy makers in the Pacific Islands region, and this poses a further challenge for developing responses (Power, Schmich & Nosa, 2015).

Harm reduction can be described as a strategy directed toward individuals or groups that aims to reduce the harms associated with certain behaviours. When applied to substance abuse, harm reduction accepts that a continuing level of alcohol and drug use (both licit and illicit) in society is inevitable and defines objectives as reducing adverse consequences. It emphasises the measurement of health, social and economic outcomes, as opposed to the measurement of drug consumption.

One approach to harm reduction would be the promotion of responsible drinking guidelines. This involves determining and communicating information about responsible and harmful levels and patterns of drinking, and how these vary in different situations and among different population groups. Examples of these guidelines are how to avoid intoxication, how to avoid long-term organic damage to the body, how to address specific population groups and information on safe, harmful and hazardous levels and patterns of consumption.

The drinking of kava is part of Pacific culture and identity, but intoxication and neglect of family and other responsibilities is not. For health reasons, kava should not be used by women who are pregnant or nursing or by patients with major mood disorders like depression. Other policies related to this approach is around restricting the availability of kava. This could occur through licensing its cultivation and/or sale, and even licensing consumption. Its price could be regulated, and it could be taxed. The number of sales outlets could be regulated, and quality control could be introduced.

Few Pacific Island countries have national drug policies and strong, well-resourced agencies responsible for their development and implementation. This policy gap means that it is difficult to implement concerted approaches to any type of drug problem in the region. The lack of data referred to above on the social and health impacts of negative substance usage is an impediment to understanding the nature of the problem and to developing interventions. In some settings one appears to be criticising, or at least cutting across, valued features of traditional and contemporary cultures when one comments about usage like kava consumption. However, the issue is to shape the policy direction through discussion in such a way that one is not, and is not seen to be, criticising traditional Pacific culture. Rather, the stance best adopted is one in which the focus is on the harm caused by some contemporary patterns of kava use, rather than on kava use as such.

PRACTICE EXAMPLE 13.1: "OPEN WORKSHEET"

The *Open Worksheet* is a talking therapy tool designed by Jioji Ravulo (Ravulo, 2009, pp. 323–327) to support the Pacific individual or group reflect on an array of topic areas, including alcohol and other drug use. The worksheet can be drawn up on any piece of paper – where on one side an oval shape is drawn with a single line underneath. On the other side, a line is drawn in the middle of the page to create two rows. Firstly, the client is asked to name a feeling that is associated with their use of alcohol and other drugs. They then draw a facial expression in the oval, with the accompanying eyes and hair to make the oval shape a picture of their face. They then write down the feeling below on the line. Afterwards, they turn the piece of paper over, and in the top section of the page, they bullet point why they feel this way about their usage. These dot points are then used to further converse and unpack verbally with the Pacific person or group their experiences, with particular attention to their thought processes and behaviours. Lastly, clients are asked to come up with some dot points as to how they can either maintain a positive approach, or more so change a negative feeling about their substance use, with a view to come up with tangible solutions and goals to effectively assist such issues. This simple dialogical tool is designed to help individuals and groups meaningfully explore their circumstances and situations, whilst taking responsibility to be part of the change process. This tool can be used with other topics, including how people feel towards their family, education, employment, significant other/partners or future.

Conclusion

Working collaboratively with Pacific people in the context of their usage is a promising sign to creating effective responses to such need. This includes meaningfully exploring why people may use certain substances, and to place this in a broader perspective. This may include understanding accessibility to such substances and the way in which certain practices are undertaken. Pacific forms of social work should be familiar with traditional and cultural views on substances to further assist strategies where usage is deemed safe, where harm minimisation is promoted and practices are undertaken within a socially defined and accepted manner and purpose.

REFLECTIVE QUESTIONS

1. What types of goals would you encourage your client to consider when trying to counteract the adverse impacts of negative substance usage?
2. How would traditional Pacific perspectives assist in promoting a harm minimisation approach?
3. Imagine you are working with Pacific teenagers – what information would you include in an educational workshop of alcohol and other drug usage?
4. There are several social factors that need to be taken into consideration when working alongside a person with a Pacific heritage background and substance use dependence. What would this include? What additional support/services would you need to consider when implementing an appropriate intervention?

References

Australian Government Department of Health. (2004). *Harm Minimisation – What is it? Module 5: Young People, Society, and AOD: Learner's Workbook*. Canberra, Austrlia: Department of Health. Retrieved from www.health.gov.au/internet/publications/publishing.nsf/Content/drugtreat-pubs-front5-wk-toc~drugtreat-pubs-front5-wk-secb~drugtreat-pubs-front5-wk-secb-6~drugtreat-pubs-front5-wk-secb-6-1

Cassileth, B. (2011). Kava (Piper methysticum). *Intergrative Oncology, 25*(4), 384–385.

Chanwai, L. G. (2000). Kava toxicity. *Emergency Medicine, 12*(2), 142–145. https://doi.org/10.1046/j.1442-2026.2000.00107.x

Devaney, M. L., Reid, G., Baldwin, S., Crofts, N. & Power, R. (2006). Illicit drug use and responses in six Pacific Island countries. *Drug and Alcohol Review, 25*(4), 387–390. https://doi.org/10.1080/09595230600741396

Faleolo, M. M. (2016). From the street to the village: The transfer of NZ youth gang culture to Sāmoa. *New Zealand Sociology, 31*(2), 48–73.

Fehoko, E. (2015). Social space and cultural identity: The faikava as a supplementary site for maintaining Tongan identity in New Zealand. *New Zealand Sociology, 30*(1), 131–139.

Glover, M., Kira, A., Min, S., Scragg, R., Nosa, V., McCool, J. & Bullen, C. (2011). Smoking is rank! But, not as rank as other drugs and bullying say New Zealand parents of pre-adolescent children. *Health Promotion Journal of Australia, 22*(3), 223–227. Retrieved from http://ezproxy.cul.columbia.edu/login?url=http://search.ebscohost.com/login. aspx?direct=true&db=cin20&AN=2011514772&site=ehost-live&scope=site

Kahn, M. W. & Fua, C. (1995). Children of South Sea Island immigrants to Australia: Factors associated with adjustment problems. *International Journal of Social Psychiatry, 41*(1), 55–73. https://doi.org/10.1177/002076409504100106

Kerr, N. (2018). Electronic cigarette usage in the Pacific. Australia: Radio Australia – Pacific Beat.

Lindstrom, L. (2009). Kava Pirates in Vanuatu? *International Journal of Cultural Property, 16*(3), 291–308. https://doi.org/10.1017/S0940739109990208

Mission Australia & Ravulo, J. (2009). *Young people and the criminal justice system: New insights and promising responses.* Sydney, Australia: Mission Australia.

Nosa, V. & Ofanoa, M. (2009). The social, cultural and medicinal use of Kava for twelve Tongan born men living in New Zealand. *Pacific Health Dialog, 15*(1), 96–102.

Nosa, V., Duffy, S., Singh, D., Lavelio, S., Amber, U., Alfred, J. & Amber, U. (2018). The use of home brew in Pacific Islands countries and territories, *Journal of Ethnicity in Substance Abuse, 17*(1), 7–15. https://doi.org/10.1080/15332640.2017.1362732

Power, R., Schmich, L. & Nosa, V. (2015). A response for substance and harm reduction in Pacific Island countries and territories. *Harm Reduction Journal, 12*(1), 10–13. https://doi.org/10.1186/s12954-015-0080-z

Quinn, B., Peach, E., Wright, C. J. C., Lim, M. S. C., Davidson, L. & Dietze, P. (2017). Alcohol and other substance use among a sample of young people in the Solomon Islands. *Australian and New Zealand Journal of Public Health, 41*(4), 358–364. https://doi.org/10.1111/1753-6405.12669

Ravulo, J. (2009). *The Development of Anti-Social Behaviour in Pacific Youth.* Sydney, Australia: University of Western Sydney.

Sam, D. L. & Berry, J. W. (2006). *The Cambridge handbook of acculturation psychology.* (D. L. Sam & J. W. Berry, Eds.). Cambridge, United Kingdom: Cambridge University Press.

Sam, D. L. & Berry, J. W. (2010). Acculturation: When individuals and groups of different cultural backgrounds meet. *Perspectives on Psychological Science, 5*(4), 472–481. https://doi.org/10.1177/1745691610373075

Schmich, L. & Power, R. (2010). *Situational analysis of drug and alcohol issues and responses in the Pacific 2008-09.* Canberra, Australia: Australian National Council on Drugs.

Secretariat of the Pacific Community. (2005). *Tobacco and alcohol in the Pacific Island Countries Trade Agreement: Impacts on population health.* Noumea, New Caledonia: Secretariat of the Pacific Community.

Shaver, J. H. & Sosis, R. (2014). How does male ritual behavior vary across the lifespan?: An examination of Fijian kava ceremonies. *Human Nature, 25*(1), 136–160. https://doi.org/10.1007/s12110-014-9191-6

Siegel, S. (2001). Pavlovian conditioning and drug overdose: When tolerance fails. *Addiction Research and Theory, 9*(5), 503–513. https://doi.org/10.3109/16066350109141767

Smith, G. B. (2011). *Kava kuo heka.* Retrieved from www.youtube.com/watch?v=qbfZAxRD8-g

Ward, C. (2001). The A, B, Cs of acculturation. In D. Matsumoto (Ed.), *The handbook of culture and psychology* (pp. 411–445). Oxford, United Kingdom: Oxford University Press.

Suggested further readings/websites

Alcohol and Drug Foundation – Drug Facts: https://adf.org.au/drug-facts/

Newcombe, D., Tanielu-Stowers, H., McDermott, R., Stephen, J., & Nosa, V. (2016). The validation of the Alcohol, Smoking and Substance Involvement Screening Test (ASSIST) among Pacific people in New Zealand, *New Zealand Journal of Psychology*, *45*(1), 30–39.

Nosa, V., Duffy, S., Singh, D., Lavelio, S., Amber, U., Homasi-Paelate, A., & Alfred, J. (2018). The use of home brew in Pacific Islands countries and territories. *Journal of Ethnicity in Substance Abuse*, *17*(1), 7–15.

Wainiqolo, I., Kool, B., Nosa, V., & Ameratunga, S. (2015). Is driving under the influence of kava associated with motor vehicle crashes? A systematic review of the epidemiological literature, *Australian and New Zealand Journal of Public Health*, *39*(5), 495–499.

14

OUR PACIFIC ELDERS AS KEEPERS AND TRANSMITTERS OF CULTURE

*Halaevalu F. Ofahengaue Vakalahi and
Ofa K.L. Hafoka-Kanuch*

Key points

- Pacific Islander elders play an integral role in the connection of past and future generations, and in the preservation of Pacific cultural values, language, rituals, ceremonies and artefacts.
- Young Pacific Islanders lean on the wisdom of their elders to help them navigate difficulties and manage dual identities.
- In Pacific cultures, inclusivity and collectivity are often demonstrated through ready access to the large extended family, social supports and intergenerational relations. Sharing, shared responsibility and interdependency are also central Pacific values that are passed down from one generation to the next through directives from the elders.

Introduction

Longevity leading to the global gerontological explosion, cultural and population shifts and worldwide migration facilitated by technology and intercultural connections warrant attention on the aging population not only because of their sheer numbers but also their significant contributions to society. As elders in Pacific communities are keepers of cultural values, language, rituals, ceremonies and artifacts (Autagavaia, 2001; Ihara & Vakalahi, 2012; Jowitt, 1990), their role is imperative in the preservation of indigenous cultural lifeways. The elders facilitate the learning of cultural values and practices that emphasise the need for connection to generations past and future (Narokobi, 1983; Ritchie & Ritchie, 1979). These elders are integral to aiding young Pacific Islanders in the diaspora in navigating life and negotiating multiple identities resulting from the immigration experience and cross cultural interactions. With an increased aging population, the cultural role of family in supporting and caring for Pacific elders has become crucial. However, with the need for individuals to relocate for employment opportunities, many families residing in rural communities are left without caregivers for the elders.

The contributions of Pacific elders to the survival of Pacific people extend beyond the pages of this chapter, however, an attempt is made to capture a few major aspects of their importance and centrality in Pacific families and communities. This chapter discusses the burgeoning needs of individuals within this developmental stage, cultural responsibilities of the Pacific elders and the duties of the families and communities to preserve the contributions of the elders relative to indigenous values, beliefs and practices. The role of social work education is also discussed in terms of educating a workforce that is ready for the challenge and thereafter the implications for research, policy and practice.

Framing the conversation

The 21st century multi-dimensional nature of Pacific identities warrants the bridging of indigenous, western and social work cultural frameworks in offering a culturally sensitive response to the needs of Pacific elders. Erikson's stages of psychosocial development (1950) describes development in middle adulthood (40–65 years) as *generativity* in which people establish careers, relationships, families and become contributing members of society, leading to the virtue of care or experience stagnation in which people are unproductive. He describes older adulthood (age 65+) as ego *integrity* in which retirement occurs, reminiscing of accomplishments and a successful life leading to the virtue of wisdom, or experience despair in which people feel guilty or regret because they did not live productive lives. For Pacific elders, the assumption is that culturally sanctioned expectations are that of generativity and integrity through contributions as navigators of their families and communities in which there is no room for failure.

In the *Ho'okele* (to navigate) model, Pacific elders are central to families and communities as keepers and transmitters of the culture (Vakalahi, Heffernan & Niu-Johnson, 2007). Connections and intergenerational relationships originate with the elders who are the spiritual links between the past, present and future. Pacific people use metaphors and symbols in their interactions and thus, a group of community elders recommended the use of the *wa'a* (canoe) as the motif for the *Ho'okele* model. The canoe symbolises the relationships among past, present and future generations as it gathers the generations and systems of the family and community. In the *Ho'okele* model, the *'akea* (hull) represents the roles and expectations of women and men with the *kane* (man) on the right side and the *wahine* (woman) on the left side or the *kapu* (sacred) side of the canoe. The *'iako* (connector) include front connectors representing the present generation and the back connectors representing past generations. Wisdom, knowledge and experiences flow from the back connectors. The *mana* (knowledge) is transmitted from the back *'iako* to the front. The *manuhope* (back end) is the most sacred part of the canoe because it represents the creation and beginning of life. Finally, the *kia* (mast) represents the connection between mortality and immortality.

The lives of Pacific elders can also be understood through an Ecological Systems Theory lens (Germain, 1979) which highlights the importance and impact of all subsystems (micro, mezzo and macro) and culture-based values, beliefs and practices. Pacific families, institutions and communities are interdependent and the effects of each of these subsystems on each other are reciprocal. The cultural, contextual and environmental aspects of a Pacific elder's life are captured as they interact interdependently with family, community, historical and cultural-based subsystems as sources of barriers and facilitators to health and wellbeing outcomes.

Integrating indigenous, western and social work frameworks can inform culturally relevant responses to the needs of Pacific elders, which will in turn allow them to lead their families and communities in ways that are relevant to present and future generations of multiple identity Pacific people. A critical component of creating culturally relevant responses to the needs of Pacific elders is the use of research methodologies that promote collaborative and inclusive participation with the community and positive outcomes. Educational curricular that prepares a relevant workforce and policies that respond to the needs of these elders are also imperative. At the core of understanding Pacific elders is a worldview of culturally sanctioned roles that spans from teacher of the culture to leader of the family. As shared by one Tongan grandmother in a study of Pacific elders in Hawai'i,

> Being a grandmother is being a mother to my grandchildren. It's more, more than being a mother, extra more doing and meaning to me as a grandmother, to love them, look after them, available to be a babysitter 24 hours (smiles), play with them, read with them. Now I try to teach my own grandchildren the language too. But I want them to know the love of the Tongan people, the respect through the way they behave, dress, and genealogy and to pass this on to their own children and grandchildren.

A Cook Island grandmother also added,

> I brought up my children in my native language but now they don't want to learn the native language, they say it's a fob language so my grandchildren don't know. So I decided when I go to school to the Kia Orana Punanga Reo, I take my grandchildren so they learn.

21st Century aging challenges for Pacific elders

Across the globe, aging comes with some broad challenges relative to lifestyle, health and mental health, care and personal endeavors. Although life expectancy is increasing in many parts of the world, many elders suffer from diseases and struggle with activities of daily living. Evidently, multiple factors contribute to the burgeoning bio-psycho-social-spiritual needs of Pacific elders. The gerontological explosion, cultural shifts, migration, technology, cross cultural connections, access to health and mental health care and other services are examples of these broader 21st century issues that impact the lives of Pacific elders and thus, their ability to act on their culturally sanctioned obligations.

Pacific elders 65+ years of age often struggle financially and incur more health problems as they age (Browne, Mokuau & Braun, 2009). Their socio-economic status becomes compromised as cost of living increases and income decreases. Health disparities increase with age if health care services are not available or accessible. Limited knowledge of available services, lack of sufficient personal resources, overcrowded housing, sparsity in culturally relevant treatment in the community and historical experiences with discrimination hinder the health and wellbeing of Pacific elders. Language barriers can also be a disincentive for seeking health and mental health services as well as transmitting the culture to a generation who do not speak the indigenous language, which can be detrimental (Sentell, Shumway & Snowden, 2007). Likewise, the digital divide in which many Pacific elders seem to be left behind because of the lack of access to technology can also be a challenge today.

Perhaps the most complex issue facing Pacific elders is mental health and illness such as depression, dementia and Alzheimer. Seeking mental health services is faced with stigma and the complexity of a spiritually grounded cultural orientation. Alzheimer's disease is a leading cause of death, memory loss, language problems and the inability to think clearly. Likewise, dementia can lead to decline in memory, communication skills and Activities of Daily Living (ADLs), which results in hallucination, aggression, agitation and danger to caregivers. Caregiving for these elders is extremely difficult under these circumstances (Schulz & Sherwood, 2008).

Many Pacific families migrate from rural home communities into cities in search for employment opportunities. The complexities of urban communities present challenges for the elders. For instance, crime, poverty and disintegrated housing often contribute to social isolation among the elders (Massey & Denton, 1993). Compounding this challenge is the overall shortage of caregivers specifically prepared to meet the demands of the aging population. This is a particular challenge for Pacific people because of the expectation that the elders are to be cared for by their families and that institutions are not necessarily a culturally acceptable option. Pacific families who live in urban communities must juggle work, family and caregiving (Yee et al., 2007).

Despite challenges, there are steps to successful aging that are universal, thus applicable to Pacific elders. According to the American Geriatrics Society (2016 www.americangeriatrics.org/) and World Health Organization (2015 www.who.int/), healthy aging requires but is not limited to: healthy habits and positive lifestyles (exercise, nutrition), keeping oneself stimulated (relationships), being careful with financial planning (retirement plan) and working to maintain dignity in old age (will). Pacific elders must be supported in successful aging in the diaspora. Technology, in particular, can facilitate availability and accessibility to healthy aging. In a study of Pacific elders in Hawai'i, one Samoan grandmother talked about her relationship with and wishes for her grandchildren,

> Relationship is 100%. I really want them to get to know their ancestors. Being a grandmother is the most humbling and beautiful experience. As a grandmother they look at you as a leader. And that would prompt you motivate you to be at your best! My grandchildren they listen to me and look at me for counselling and sometimes they'll say to their parents "oh but nana said to do this". I love that because I was raised by my grandparents. We were brought up to speak the truth, to be honest you don't go and get things from other people's place, and if you do, you go and give it back. I've instilled that in my grandchildren, and be kind and help one another, these are some of the things that my grandfather was a planter and he give things to everybody and I've developed that. I've taught my children my church, the gospel, the word of wisdom.

Indigenous Pacific culture and the elders

Pacific elders bridge the generations by cultivating indigenous cultural values while facilitating the embracing of the "new" cultural values by their posterity (Ihara & Vakalahi, 2012). Regardless of time or space, Pacific elders are highly respected as central to the survival of Pacific cultures through serving as teachers and navigators of their families and communities (Vakalahi, Heffernan & Niu Johnson, 2007). They teach, carry out traditions and pass on cultural ceremonies, rituals, customs and protocols to the upcoming generation (Autagavaia, 2001; Taufe'ulungaki, 2008; Vakalahi & Godinet, 2014; Vakalahi, Ihara & Hafoka, 2014; Westervelt, 1910). For example, inclusivity and collectivity are often demonstrated through ready access to the large extended family, social supports and intergenerational relations. Sharing, shared responsibility and interdependency are also central Pacific values that are passed down from one generation to the next through directives from the elders (McDermott, Tsêng, & Maretzki, 1980; Mokuau, 1991; Vakalahi & Godinet, 2014).

Worldwide migration, which results in dual and multiple cultural identities, and transnational identities have also emerged as critical issues for Pacific elders (Fong & Furuto, 2001). The elders assist the young in navigating these identities and negotiating cultural conflicts. For instance, individualistic decision making conflicts with the collective decision making nature of Pacific cultures in which the family and/or community have a role. Likewise, navigating the responsibility of the young to care for the elders often requires the wisdom of the collective. Placing an elder in a nursing or group home is not an easy option in collectivist Pacific cultures (Long & Long, 1982; McLaughlin & Braun, 1998).

Intergenerational life as an inherent part of Pacific cultures has contributed positively to linking generations, transmitting cultural values and practices and the survival of Pacific people, particularly in industrialised societies (Banks, 2009; Dodd, 1990; Senyürekli & Detzner, 2008; Waites, 2008). Through an intergenerational context, the codes of conduct such as respect for the elders and women, reciprocity, collectivity, spirituality and ceremonies and rituals are preserved and passed on to the young. This shared space facilitates a strong cultural foundation upon which the young can build their lives, particularly Pacific people with multi-cultural identities (Vakalahi, Heffernan & Niu Johnson, 2007). The collective nature of Pacific cultures relative to unconditional love, loyalty, respect, reciprocity and shared meaning and responsibility contributes to the preservation of this practice (Tamasese, Peteru, Waldegrave & Bush, 2005). In parenting, investment is in kin and community and shared trust and responsibility for all children. Intergenerational living stems beyond economic necessities, suggesting that a child has a collective purpose and connection to all living across generations (Ritchie, 1979). It is the sacred responsibility of the elders to lead and ensure cultural continuity through linking generations (Kenney, 1976; Laville & Berkowitz, 1944). In return, Pacific families and communities must support the elders in all dimensions of their lives and specifically in caregiving, finances and health care. Of great significance today is the need for indigenous medicine as an option available for Pacific elders.

Pacific approaches and strategies

Effective strategies are often defined by the target culture, thus incorporating Pacific epistemologies in community work, practice, policy and research is imperative. A few prominent approaches and strategies are described as follows.

The Pacific Conceptual Framework (Ministry of Social Development, New Zealand Government [2012]) was created in Aotearoa New Zealand by and for Pacific people based on inclusivity, collectivity, reciprocity and interdependency and promotes family wellbeing. It is grounded on the following frameworks: Turanga Māori (Cook Islands); Vuvale Doka Sautu (Fijian); Koe Fakatupuolamaoui he tau Magafaoua Niu (Niuean); le tōfā mamao (Samoan); Toku fou Tiale (Tuvalu); Fofola e fala kae talanoa e kainga (Tongan); and Kāiga Māopoopo (Tokelauan). Fundamental components of the framework include: family is central; language is critical; rituals and relationships contribute to wellbeing; and ethnic-specific practice is imperative (Ministry of Social Development, New Zealand Government [2012]). Other indigenous approaches also include: Ifoga (Jantzi, 2001) Samoan reconciliation practice; Fakalelei (Jantzi, 2001) Tongan practice; Pola and Uku (Mafile'o, 2005) community practice; Seitapu (Pulotu-Endemann, Suaali'i-Sauni et al., 2007) mental health practice; Family Group Conferencing (Wilcox et al., 1991); E Kaveinga (Crummer et al., 1998) child welfare; Fonofale (Pulotu-Endemann, 2002); Ho'oponopono

(Pukui, Haertig & Lee, 1972) conflict resolution; and Popao (Fotu & Tafa, 2009) cultural identity.

In examining and determining the most relevant approaches and strategies for Pacific elders, professionals must consider the following: history and context; culturally and linguistically competent professionals; multi-cultural and multi-generational influence, transnationalism and transcultural experiences; family and community as origins of socialisation; and the role of spirituality. In a study on Pacific elders in Hawai'i, a Native Hawaiian grandmother shared her indigenous perspective,

> We know that if you ate poi instead of rice it's a good thing and the doctor restated the fact that poi if you ate it every day it is one of the best medicines. The Hawaiian the Polynesian way of eating, the best way, you have taro, ulu, fa'i, maia. Poi is expensive but if we took a bag of poi it would be better than running for fast food and it's cheaper in the long run ... just starting to get back to our basics. Right now I have a cold in my right eye and one of the things that I remember my grandma would dab certain leaves for boils, popoa leafs ... and put it on my eye and this swelling right here will go down. The culture is still alive in us still lives in us, "aloe" that's one of the things I plant in my own garden. Growing up we were seldom sick because grandparents knew what to do for us. We can get back some of our cultural ways drinking noni, guavas for all the different reasons. When you know you doing something right it just makes you a right person. One of the best medicines is to be outward to other people ... psychologically that is the best it just makes you feel better it makes you glow inside. Our ancestors, the ocean, that's the medicine the Lord gave to us, Akua, you look at the mountains you know and for my own well-being it's talking to you right in my na'au, it's a medicine earth. Now my Polynesian upbringing is you put that flower on because you become that flower that's a Polynesian thing, your laughter you cannot bottle it up, it's gotta go out in order to come back in and if you cannot sing, sing anyway because you know the Akua does not hear flat he only hears what you want to share.

Implications for social work

The role of social work education as a precursor for culturally relevant social work practice is critical to educating a workforce that is ready for the challenge and the implications for research, policy and practice relative to Pacific elders and elders across cultures. For instance, social work curriculum must include content on gerontology for both undergraduate and postgraduate levels. The classroom must offer effective teaching and learning strategies in Pacific social and community work. Social work as a profession must acknowledge the implications for social work education and training in the Pacific region. Professional social work organisations across the globe must have statements on aging, gerontology and geriatrics. Field education must consider providing experiences that lead to graduates who are workforce ready for the global gerontological explosion.

In all, social work must create spaces that allow for dialogues about questions such as: What are the impacts of colonisation and immigration on multiple identities? What culturally relevant assessment tools can be used for effectively working with Pacific elders? What are the culturally and linguistically informed services available specifically for Pacific elders? What is the role of cultural strengths in working with Pacific elders? What are the strategies for positioning the issues of Pacific elders in the global conversations? The case of Moana suggested a few lessons learned:

CASE STUDY 14.1

Moana is an immigrant Tongan American great grandfather. He lives with his wife on the Northshore of 'Oahu in the State of Hawai'i. He was a teacher and middle school principal of 20 years in Tonga. He migrated with his family to the U.S. in 1977 to attend college. In Hawai'i, he worked in the Polynesian Cultural Center until retirement. He is bilingual, but more fluent in the Tongan language. He is active physically and socially, facilitated by the warm weather of Hawai'i and the support of families and friends. In 2013, while on a trip to Utah, Moana was admitted to the emergency room and thereafter admitted to the hospital for surgery to remove a tumor which event led to decreased functionality and inability to perform basic Activities of Daily Living (ADLs). He experienced extreme weight loss from the radiation, constant pain and pain medication, and disorientation and psychological stress from being dependent on others for basic ADLs. Upon discharge from the hospital, Moana's health turned for the worst being unable to feed himself and attend to his personal hygiene. He needed professional physical therapy. His family had to make a decision about caregiving. "Taking care of our own" was the Pacific way thus placing an elder in a facility is unacceptable. Challenges were also posed by the fact that his children did not live in close proximity. Thus there was a need to consider an integration of Pacific and western perspectives, a hybrid model of caregiving which facilitated caring from a distance. His wife became his primary caregiver and children were secondary caregivers contributing support in housing and finances. Travel and technological advances facilitated iphone Face-Time with family as well as opportunities to "talk stories", take his temperature, clean his room, run errands, etc.

Overall, a hybrid model allowed the integration of Pacific culture and the realities of American life. For professionals, first, provide cultural competency training particularly for the aged and those from cultures that are different. Second, for elders from a different culture, the head/lead physician needs to take the time to visit and follow up. Third, a comprehensive treatment plan is critical for elders, especially those with a new terminal illness diagnosis and those undergoing surgery. Fourth, discharge requires the presence of the lead providers in order to avoid miscommunication and misunderstanding and the appearance of negligence. Fifth, an elder who had surgery should not be pushed out prematurely; they heal slower in body and emotions. Lastly, communication, communication, communication; follow up follow up follow up for a positive experience in the health care system. Keeping the patient and his/her family informed is crucial. Moving forward, social work as a profession must collectively lift and leverage their wide range of expertise to cultivate culturally and linguistically relevant responses to the multi-dimensional needs of elders across cultures and in this case, Pacific elders. Preservation of Pacific cultural values and practices are crucial for the survival of Pacific people in the disapora and Pacific elders are the helm.

References

Autagavaia, M. (2001). Social Work with Pacific Island Communities. In Connolly, M. (ed.), *New Zealand Social Work: Contexts and Practice*, pp. 72–84. Melbourne, Australia: Oxford University Press.

Banks, S. P. (2009). Intergenerational ties across borders: Grandparenting narratives by expatriate retirees in Mexico, *Journal of Aging Studies*, 23(3), 178–187.

Browne, C. V., Mokuau, N. & Braun, K. L. (2009). Adversity and resiliency in the lives of Native Hawaiian elders. *Social Work*, 54(3), 253–261.

Crummer, A., Samuel, M., Papai-Vao, T. & George, C. (1998). *E Kaveinga: A Cook Islands model of social work practice*. Wellington, New Zealand: Children, Young Persons and Their Families Service.

Dodd, E. (1990). *The Island world of Polynesia*. Putney, VT: Windmill Hill Press.

Erikson, E. (1950). *Childhood and society* (1st ed.). New York: Norton

Fong, R. & Furuto, S. M. (Eds.). (2001). *Culturally competent practice: Skills, interventions, and evaluations*. New York: Pearson College Division.

Fotu, M. & Tafa, T. (2009). The Popao Model: A Pacific recovery and strength concept in mental health. *Pacific Health Dialogue*, 15(1), 164–170.

Germain, C. (1979). "Ecology and social work". In *Social work practice: People and environments*. Edited by: Germain, C. (pp. 1–22). New York: Columbia University Press.

Ihara, E. S. & Vakalahi, H. F. O. (2012). Collective worldviews and health: Through the lens of Pacific American elders. *Journal of Educational Gerontology*, 38(6), 400–411.

Jantzi, V. E. (2001). *Restorative justice in New Zealand: Current practice, future possibilities*. Retrieved from www.massey.ac.nz/~wtie/articles/vern.htm.

Jowitt, G. (1990). *Church going in the Pacific*. Auckland, New Zealand: Longman Paul Limited.

Kenney, M. (1976). *Youth in Micronesia in the 1970s: The impact of changing family, employment, and justice systems*, Washington, DC: U.S. Department of Justice for the Community Development Division of the Public Affairs Department of the Trust Territory of the Pacific Islands.

Laville, J. & Berkowitz, J. (1944). *Pacific Island legends: Life and legends in the South Pacific Islands*. Noumea, New Caledonia: Librarie Pentecost.

Long, S. & Long, B. (1982). Curable cancers and fatal ulcers: Attitudes toward cancer in Japan. *Social Science and Medicine*, 16(24), 2101–2108.

Mafile'o, T. A. (2005). *Tongan metaphors of social work practice: Hangē ha Pā kuo Fa'u'* (Doctoral dissertation). Massey University, Palmerston North, New Zealand. Available from Massey Research Online at: http://hdl.handle.net/10179/1697

Massey, D. S. & Denton, N. A. (1993). *American apartheid: Segregation and the making of the underclass.* Cambridge, MA: Harvard University Press.

McDermott, J. F. Jr., Tseng, W. & Maretzki, T. W. (1980). *People and cultures of Hawaii: A psychocultural profile.* Honolulu, HI: The University Press of Hawaii.

McLaughlin, L. A. & Braun, K. L. (1998). Asian and Pacific Islander cultural values: Considerations for health care decision making. *Health & Social Work, 23*(2), 116–126.

Ministry of Social Development, New Zealand Government (2012). Nga vaka o kāiga tapu: A Pacific Conceptual Framework to address family violence in New Zealand. Retrieved from http://pasefikaproud.co.nz/assets/Resources-for-download/PasefikaProudResource-Nga-Vaka-o-Kaiga-Tapu-Main-Pacific-Framework.pdf

Mokuau, N. (Ed.). (1991). *Handbook of social services for Asian and Pacific Islanders.* New York, NY: Greenwood.

Narokobi, B. (1983). *The Melanesian way.* Suva, Fiji: Institute of Pacific Island Studies, University of the South Pacific.

Pukui, M. K., Haertig, E. W. & Lee, C. A. (1972). Nānā i ke Kumu: Look to the Source, vol. 1. Honolulu, HI: Hui Hānai.

Pulotu-Endemann, K. F. (2002). *Consequences of alcohol and other drug use: Fonofale.* Retrieved from www.alcohol.org.nz/resources/publications/ALAC_drug_Manual_Chapter_4.pdf

Pulotu-Endemann, F. K., Suaali'i-Sauni, T., Lui, D., McNicholas, T., Milne, M. & Gibbs, T. (2007). *Seitapu Pacific mental health and addiction cultural & clinical competencies framework.* Auckland: The National Centre of Mental Health Research and Workforce Development.

Ritchie, J. (1979). *Growing up in Polynesia.* North Sydney, New South Wales: National Library of Australia.

Ritchie J. & Ritchie, J. (1979). *Growing up in Polynesia.* North Sydney, New South Wales: National Library of Australia.

Schulz, R. & Sherwood, P. R. (2008). Physical and mental health effects of family caregiving. *Journal of Social Work Education, 44*(3), 105–113.

Sentell, T., Shumway, M. & Snowden, L. (2007). Access to mental health treatment by English language proficiency and race/ethnicity. *Journal of General Internal Medicine, 22*(2), 289–293.

Senyurekli, A. R. & Detzner, D. F. (2008). Intergenerational Relationships in a Transnational Context: The Case of Turkish Families. *Family Relations, 57*(4), 457–467.

Tamasese, K., Peteru, C. & Waldegrave, C. (2005). Ole Taeao Afua, the new morning: A qualitative investigation into Samoan perspectives on mental health and culturally appropriate services. *The Australian and New Zealand Journal of Psychiatry, 39*(4), 300–309.

Taufe'ulungaki, A. (2008). "Fonua": Reclaiming Pacific communities in Aotearoa. Conference presentation, LotuMoui. Auckland, New Zealand: Counties-Manukau District Health Board.

Vakalahi, H. F. O. & Godinet, M. (2014). *Transnational Pacific Islander Americans and social work: Dancing to the beat of a different drum.* Washington, DC: NASW Press.

Vakalahi, H. F. O., Heffernan, K. & Niu Johnson, R. (2007). Pacific Island elderly: A model for bridging generations and systems. *The Journal of Baccalaureate Social Work, 12*(2), 26–41.

Vakalahi, H.F.O., Ihara, E.S. & Hafoka, M.P. (2014). Family roots: Sustenance for Samoan and Tongan American elders. *Journal of Family Strengths, 13*(1), 1–17.

Waites, C. (2008). *Social work practice with African-American families: An intergenerational perspective.* New York: Routledge.

Westervelt, W. D. (1910). *Legends of Maui – A Demi God of Polynesia and of his mother Hina.* Honolulu, HI: The Hawaiian Gazette Co., LTD.

Wilcox, R., Smith, D., Moore, J., Hewitt, A., Allan, G., Walker, H. ... Featherstone, T. (1991). *Family decision making & family group conference.* Lower Hutt, New Zealand: Practitioners' Publishing.

Yee, B. W. K., DeBaryshe, B. D., Yuen, S., Kim, S. Y. & McCubbin, H. I. (2007). Asian American and Pacific Islander families: Resiliency and life-span socialization in a cultural context. In F. T. L. Leong, A. G. Inman, A. Ebreo, L. H Yang, L. Kinoshita, & M. Fu (eds.), *Handbook of Asian American psychology* (pp. 69–86, 2nd ed.). Thousand Oaks, CA: Sage.

15
UNDERSTANDING SEXUAL AND GENDER DIVERSITY IN THE PACIFIC ISLANDS

Geir Henning Presterudstuen

Key points

- LGBTQI+ people are subject to various forms of discrimination throughout the Pacific Islands region.
- Sexual relations between men are effectively still criminalised in seven countries in the region, and de facto legal protection of LGBTQI+ people are limited in many others.
- Different Pacific Island communities have different gender ideologies and various traditions of non-heteronormative people and gender variance.
- Social workers need to be cautious about applying social, political, theoretical or analytical concepts of the Euro-American tradition when trying to understand non-heteronormative people and communities in the Pacific Islands.

Introduction

The overall global pattern in the circumstances for LGBTQI+[1] individuals is one of increased visibility and political representation and improved recognition of minority rights. Decriminalisation of same-sex practices and legal recognition of same-sex relationships are significantly more widespread now than in recent history. Still, according to the International Lesbian, Gay, Bisexual, Trans and Intersex Association (ILGA, 2017), various degrees of same-sex relations remain criminalised in 72 countries across the globe and many other states fail to offer full legal protection or recognition of non-heteronormative minorities.[2] In most contexts, LGBTQI+ peoples are at increased risks of a number of social and economic stress indicators, including those associated with health outcomes and economic security. Limited legal protection and adverse socio-economic outcomes are particularly common in parts of the global south.

It is also true that current discourses about LGBTQI+ rights remain largely driven by and centred on the global north in ways that fail to take into account the true cultural diversity of non-heteronormative individuals and groups globally. The relatively narrow focus on human rights and legal recognition in context of such demands as same-sex marriage has facilitated an increased homogenisation of LGBTQI+ identities and demands in ways that privilege urban, Anglo-American cultural, social and economic contexts over others. LGBTQI+ people in cultural regions like the Pacific Islands, for instance, often struggle to gain recognition for their culturally specific gender and sexual identities within such discourses.

PACIFIC TERMINOLOGY

Fa'afafine (Samoa, America Samoa and Tokelau), *Fakaleiti* or *Leiti* (Tonga), *Fakafifine* (Niue), *Akava'ine* or *laelae* (Cook Islands), *Mahu* (Tahiti and Hawaii), *Vakasalewalewa* (Fiji), *Palopa* (PNG), *Tangata ira tane* (NZ Māori) are all terms used by Pasifika trans people to self-identify but their precise meaning is best understood in the cultural contexts they emerge.

Qauri (Fiji) is a term used to describe a variety of non-heteronormative people in Fiji. Often translated as "gay" to English speakers the true meaning of *qauri* can range from derogatory to endearing depending on who utilises it. Similar words, often based on localised versions of English language terms, can be found across the region. NZ Māori uses the more value-neutral term *Takatāpui* to refer to an intimate companion of the same sex (also in use in Cook Islands and Tokelau).

LGBTQI+ in the Pacific Islands: The legal context

Pacific Island communities have a long tradition of gender variance and the inclusion of non-heteronormative social performers in the gender system. While many of these are becoming increasingly visible in the modern service economy of urban centres across the region, the social acceptance of non-heteronormativity is also mediated by a number of social, religious, political and cultural factors. From a social work point of view, it is worth noting that gender variance in itself might often be a risk factor for social exclusion, discrimination, socio-economic disadvantage and a number of health risks through the Pacific Islands. In many instances, they are also explicitly targeted by legislation.

In the Pacific Islands region, seven countries still effectively criminalise sexual relations between men under the guise of prohibition against "sodomy", "acts against nature" or "indecency". Those countries are Cook Islands,[3] Kiribati,

Papua New Guinea (PNG), Samoa, Solomon Islands, Tonga and Tuvalu. Additionally, the Solomon Islands also explicitly prohibits "indecent practices" between all people of the same sex. If proven, committing, or allowing other people to commit these acts on oneself, might lead to imprisonment for between 3 and 14 years depending on the legal context. In Tonga, any person convicted of "sodomy" or "bestiality" might also be sentenced to whipping in addition to imprisonment.[4] Despite recent international pressure to decriminalise same-sex acts to bring local legislation more in line with global trends in human rights and protection for sexual minorities, political and judicial forces in these countries consistently use forms of cultural defence to maintain the legal persecution of same-sex relations.

Although some countries in the region has recently decriminalised same-sex relations, namely Vanuatu (2007), Fiji (2013), Palau (2014) and Nauru (2016), and broader anti-discrimination laws in general cover sexual minorities, de facto legal protection and social acceptance varies significantly between and within these countries. Same-sex unions or marriages are, for instance, neither legalised nor recognised in any of the independent countries of the region (but have been legally recognised in all foreign territories in the region since 2017 except Cook Islands, Niue and Tokelau [New Zealand territories] and Easter Island [Chilean territory]). The limitations of legal protection for sexual minorities even in these locales is illustrated by, for instance, how Fiji's Prime Minister, Frank Bainimarama, who has otherwise cultivated a progressive persona in regional and international politics, labelled same-sex marriage "rubbish" that would never be legalised in his lifetime.[5] This highlights the complexity of LGBTQI+'s experience of legal protection in fear of persecution in the Pacific Islands.

For social work practitioners, this legal context represents particular challenges. Given many laws and policies, including those aimed at protecting individuals from violence, discrimination and persecution, in reality excludes LGBTQI+ individuals the commitment to support and value these communities, as well as social equality more broadly, implies working against local legal framework as advocates and allies. Some organisations that in other contexts might be considered natural working partners, including faith-based organisations and public service agencies, might also be resistant to provide support for LGBTQI+ individuals.

CASE STUDY 15.1: SAME-SEX RELATIONSHIP

Ruth and Sara have recently moved out of their respective villages in the Papua New Guinean Highlands to live together in Port Moresby. Both had experienced verbal abuse and threats in their villages after their same-sex relationship had become common knowledge. They no longer feel they can fully rely on the support from their kinship networks although they still keep in contact with some close family. They hoped life in town would provide more privacy and independence but recently they have been targeted by members of a local ministry who have harassed them in public and threatened to report them to the police for sexual perversion.

What initial advice would you provide to Ruth and Sara in addressing their fear of being reported to the police and their general safety?

What are some cultural considerations you would consider when providing professional support for Ruth and Sara?

What possible resources do you think they could access locally?

The historical and cultural context

Underlying this legal context is a historical and cultural complexity surrounding non-heteronormativity, gender fluidity and various forms of same-sex relations that varies significantly from community to community and makes generalisations across the region difficult. Traditionally, many communities in the Pacific Islands had ways of talking about and understanding sexual development and diversity that were more permissive than what one might find in the global north even today. Early colonials and researchers found their Western middle class moralities shaken by the extent and level of sexual innuendo and jokes in the communities they encountered. One prominent case is the famous anthropologist Bronislaw Malinowski who reportedly blushed in embarrassment over the frankness with which Trobriand islanders (in PNG) brought issues about sexuality into everyday conversations. The same might have been true throughout the Pacific region, and it is fair to assume that much of what is emphasised as "traditional" local sexual morality today is just as much a product of Christianisation and the consolidation of patriarchal power that followed the colonial project as any deep-seated local beliefs.

A common trope associated with LGBTQI+ issues in the research of highlands Papua New Guinea and other parts of Melanesia, for instance, was the notion of ritualised homosexuality. Popularised by the work of anthropologist Gilbert Herdt (1981; 1984) and later taken up by a number of other researchers (cf. Ernst 1991; Knauft 2003), ritualised homosexuality became a catch-all term for a variety of gender and initiation rites found throughout Melanesia that included exchange of semen, mutual masturbation and fellatio. Looking at these practices through the notion of ritualised homosexuality effectively created a framework for cross-cultural studies of homosexual practices that took western definitions of sex and sexuality as yardsticks. A key problem with this is the proclivity to employ a modern, Euro-American viewpoint to label practices "sexual" that are not perceived as such locally. In the context of the semen rituals described by Herdt and others, it is now obvious that thinking of them in terms of sex and sexuality provides little of analytical value. They served important functions in male-to-male sociality and particularly the initiation of young men into adulthood but there is no evidence participants engaged in regular or long-term same-sex relations.

At the same time, an over-emphasis of these ritual forms led to widespread ignorance of sexual diversity in Melanesia more broadly. Bruce Knauft, who has conducted long-term fieldwork among the Gebusi in PNG, observed that this community "exemplified a diverse and overlapping range of heterosexualities, homosexualities, and bisexualities" (Knauft, 2003, pp. 141–142) that were common across Melanesia. That implies that local traditions embraced a wide variety of sexual traditions and norms, and many communities included same-sex practices that were not ritualised and that existed outside age-structured relationships described by Herdt.

Still, throughout Melanesia these ritual practices have largely disappeared and become anathema to good moral behaviour post-Christianisation. This process was perhaps made easier by the fact that most same-sex practices became intrinsically linked to pre-modern rituals rather than a broader tradition of sexual diversity in the colonial imagination. Bruce Knauft moreover observed that many of his young participants among the Gebusi in PNG appeared to have no knowledge of the same-sex practices of their relatively recent ancestors. It is also telling that local LGBTQI+ activists make no reference to earlier ritual practices in their claims for decriminalisation of same-sex practices and relationships.

Elsewhere in the Pacific, the popular discourse around gendered and sexual diversity has to a large extent been framed by the concept of "third gender". Such a notion is most prominently attached to gender liminal identity categories like the Samoan *fa'afafine*, *māhū* in Hawaii, Tongan *fakaleiti* and *laelae* in the Cook Islands. These are all well-established and socially recognised categories of people who fail to fit within the gender binary model of (masculine) men and (feminine) women but can instead be described as male-bodied transgender people. Their prevalence and the relative acceptance of them in their respective societies, particularly but not exclusively throughout Polynesia, led to them frequently being defined as a separate, third gender category that existed in the region and elsewhere[6] in many early colonial and scientific accounts, while in contemporary society they are often considered to be local variations of same-sex attracted identities such as gay or homosexual.

In reality, however, individuals self-identifying or labelled with these identity markers belie easy categorisations in Euro-American gender/sexuality terms. In Fiji, for instance, a wide variation of non-heteronormative social performers ranging from cross-dressers and transgender to presumably masculine performing males that engage in same-sex practices are often grouped together under the local term *qauri*. Derogatory in origin, the term *qauri* is commonly translated as poofter, fag, gay, queen or homosexual depending on context and intention of the speaker but is also widely used as a term of self-identification for a variety of same-sex oriented persons. Similarly, in her discussion of the *laelae* of the

Cook Islands, Kalissa Alexeyeff argues that they belong to a "category of feminised masculinity that is common throughout the Pacific" and refer to a great number of different practices and identity traits, from "women trapped in men's bodies" to presumably heterosexual men with female friends and white-collar jobs to cross-dressers and boys wearing men's clothes, lipstick and female jewellery (2008, p. 147). More striking, however, is the construction of *laelae* as a sexual category:

> A key difference between *laelae* and Western homosexuals is that self-identified *laelae* sexually desire straight men, not other *laelae*. *Laelae* I spoke to found the idea of having sexual relations with another *laelae* as largely incomprehensible and likened it to sleeping with someone of the same sex. Straight men who have sex with *laelae* are not considered, and do not consider themselves, to be homosexual.
>
> *(Alexeyeff, 2008, p. 147)*

This is neither a typically South Pacific phenomenon, nor is it new. In fact, the understanding of sexual relationships as existing on a strict binary line with hetero- and homosexual appears to be a fairly recent creation:

> The most striking difference between the dominant sexual culture of the early twentieth century and that of our own era is the degree to which the earlier culture permitted men to engage in sexual relations with other men, often on a regular basis, without requiring them to regard themselves – or be regarded by others – as gay ... Many men ... neither understood nor organized their sexual practices along a hetero-homosexual axis.
>
> *(Chauncey, 1995, p. 65)*

In the Pacific Islands, this must also be understood in relation to the cultural constructions of self which often differ greatly from their Western equivalents. It is gender, rather than sexual identity, that is given ontological priority in the wider Pacific region, and gender liminal identities, as with all other social identities, are mainly defined with respect to their role in social life and centred on their expected contribution to collective life as opposed to inner, personal desires (Alexeyeff, 2008; Besnier, 1994). To equate these traditional notions of gender liminality with a Western understanding of gayness and homosexuality is consequently a simplification, although it is clear that modern appropriations of "third genders" are often equated with a same-sex orientation by society at large in many contexts of the Pacific.[7]

The contemporary context

The advent of modern life and the emergence of Western social institutions and practices obviously engineered a redefinition of many social categories throughout the Pacific, and this is perhaps particularly true for those on the margin of the traditional structure. In the contemporary Pacific, as well as elsewhere, the meanings assigned to being non-heteronormative or same-sex oriented subjects are dynamically shaped and reshaped under the conditions of globalisation and westernisation and local subjects are often redefined and reconstructed in relation to what Dennis Altman has famously labelled a "global gay identity" (1997). This is a process of internationalisation of not only the cultural and aesthetic markers of "gayness" – from films, magazines, fashion, music and corporeal performance – but also the relatively recent and distinctly Anglo-American emphasis on same-sex desire as the key aspect of non-heteronormative identities independent of gender identity. Throughout the Pacific this is evident in how local forms of non-heteronormativity are combined with, challenged by or in some cases substituted by an increasingly popular global gay identity which is "no longer considered an expression of 'really' being a woman in a man's body (or vice versa), but rather as physically desiring others of one's own gender without necessarily wishing to deny one's masculinity/femininity" (Altman, 2001, p. 26).

What becomes clear amidst this socio-cultural change is that the romantic view about the apparent widespread tolerance for homoeroticism and non-heteronormativity in Pacific Island traditions has at the same time disguised various forms of persecution and violence against sexual and gendered minorities. Presterudstuen has demonstrated how the relative social acceptance of *qauri* in traditional Fiji has long been premised upon a denial of their rights to sexual agency and a cultural practice of unmarried men using them for sexual favours (2014; 2019). Schmidt (2010) similarly argues that the exoticisation and eroticisation of *fa'afafine* stems from a long research tradition, starting with Margaret Mead's controversial *Coming of Age in Samoa* (1928), that has over-emphasised sexual frivolity and ignored the ongoing marginalisation of women and non-heteronormative people in Samoa.

What is more, while modernity and urban life is often perceived to be offering new opportunities for self-realisation and personal freedom for gender variant people, the reality is often different. The increase of fundamental Christianity across the region has put pressure on many traditional forms, ideas, rituals and practices including those pertaining to gender and sexual identities. Christian moralities are often used explicitly to target non-heteronormative individuals both judicially and extra-judicially and to justify persecution of gender variant individuals. In Papua New Guinea, for instance, homophobic violence and hate crimes are frequently reported.[8] In fact, across the region, evidence suggests that developing new sexual and gendered identities outside the highly regulated social systems of traditional institutions has frequently led to increased social isolation and persecution for non-heteronormative subjects in many Pacific communities. Fijian *qauri* leaving their villages for more freedom to express their own sexualities often face economic difficulties and social isolation in Fijian cities (Presterudstuen, 2014; 2019). Similar dynamics have been pointed out in Samoa where *fa'afafine* are increasingly victimised and subjected to religious persecution, discrimination, violence and exploitation. In fact, this pattern is evident throughout the region where gender and sexually diverse populations are at significantly higher risks of contracting sexually transmitted infections, including HIV/AIDS, and becoming victims of violence, partly associated with their over-representation in sex work.

> **CASE STUDY 15.2: POSSIBLE PROBLEMS WITH DATA COLLECTION**
>
> As part of a programme on sexual health funded by an international aid organisation, you are asked to help identify the extent to which local LGBTQI+ people engage in sex work in urban centres in Fiji and Tonga. In the research material you are provided, individuals you work with are asked to identify as "Gay", "Lesbian", "Queer" or "Other".
>
> Reflect upon some of the possible problems with this exercise.
>
> How would you utilise your cultural consideration and competency to improve the process of data collecting?

Although the dynamics described above are common risk factors for non-heteronormative individuals across the world, open discrimination and social exclusion have another layer in the Pacific Islands that is crucial for social workers to keep in mind. The collectivist nature of Pacific Island communities and the strong connection people generally have not only to their extended families and kinship networks but also their ancestral land creates significant emotional difficulties for people that become removed from their community. As a consequence, many are likely to endure significant persecution before they willingly remove themselves from their kinship network. Those becoming displaced from their communities often harbour conflicting emotions to their kinship networks on top of suffering materially from being removed from local cycles of reciprocity and responsibility.

Activists and scholars have highlighted that the relatively vulnerable position of non-heteronormative individuals in the Pacific Islands must be seen in context of the widespread patriarchal nature of these societies. Although there is local and regional variance, most Pacific Islands cultures are based on patrilocal family units with male authority and male lines of descent, while women, children and non-heteronormative subjects are relatively subordinate.

It is also worth noting that in contrast to the relative ubiquity of same-sex oriented or transgender males, females that challenge gender binaries are comparatively invisible in Pacific Island communities. Although, as discussed earlier, same-sex practices between women are not specifically outlawed anywhere except the Solomon Islands, intimate relationships between women are rarely culturally

TABLE 15.1 Glossary of terms used within Chapter

LGBTQI+:	This term includes Lesbian, Gay, Bisexual, Trans, Queer, Intersex and other non-heteronormative gender or sexual identities people may subscribe to.
Gender:	The social and cultural construction of what it means to be a man, woman or some other term, including ideologies, roles, expectations and behaviour.
Sex:	A medically defined term, usually categorising a person as "male" or "female" (or indeterminate sex) based on their biological make-up (their reproductive functions and chromosomes).
Intersex:	A general term used for a variety of conditions in which a person is born with reproductive or sexual anatomy that does not seem to fit the typical biological definitions of female or male. Some people now self-identify as "intersex", while many people who are intersex or have an intersex medical condition identify simply as male or female. Intersex is thus a distinct category from trans-identities, and the majority of trans-people are not born with intersex medical conditions.
Transgender:	A person whose gender identity is different from their physical sex at birth.
Transsexual:	A person who has changed, or is in the process of changing, their sex to conform to their gender identity.
Cross-dresser:	A person who wears the clothing and/or accessories considered by society to correspond to another gender.
Gay:	Today gay is used to describe the sexual orientation and cultural expression of people of all genders who self-identify as same-sex attracted. The term emerged in British English and was popularised by homosexual men in the 1960s American counter-culture movement and does not have a universal meaning worldwide.
Non-heteronormative:	Heteronormativity is the ideology that all human beings naturally fall into one out of two binary gender categories (men/women) and that sexual relations naturally go across these (heterosexuality), thus aligning biological sex, gender identity, gender performance and sexual identity. Everyone whose gender performance, sexual identities or sexual relationships divert from and challenge this can be viewed as 'non-heteronormative'.

recognised. One possible exception is the category of tomboys in Samoa that are constructed in opposition to *fa'afafine*. However, just like their opposites, tomboys are broadly seen as a gender category, that is, female-bodied persons that come to be viewed as behaving "like men" and take on social responsibilities predominantly associated with boys and men at a certain stage in life, rather than a sexual identity, and there is little social acceptance of their sexual agency.

Conclusion

When working with individuals that self-identify, or are identified by others, as non-heteronormative, it is crucial to acknowledge the many ways in which various societal and social influences, including different forms of oppression and discrimination, impact these clients as well as the broader communities served. One must also be aware that these dynamics might differ significantly from community to community. In practical terms, that means that social workers need to gain profound cultural competency in the specific community in which they work and be sensitive to culturally specific, local ideologies, beliefs and power dynamics pertaining to gender and sexuality.

This becomes particularly acute in the Pacific Islands where there is significant cultural diversity in perceptions of same-sex relationships and intimacies and where the social issues they face are consequently varied across communities. The examples above also demonstrate how LGBTQI+ identities in the region are also deeply rooted in the specifics of local histories and gender ideologies. A consequence of this is that we need to be cautious about applying social, political, theoretical or analytical concepts of the Euro-American tradition when trying to understand non-heteronormative people and communities in the Pacific Islands.

Notes

1 This term includes Lesbian, Gay, Bisexual, Trans, Queer, Intersex and other non-heteronormative gender or sexual identities people may subscribe to. In this chapter, I use this and 'non-heteronormative' interchangeably as descriptive, catch-all terms for the diverse communities and individuals framed by my analysis.
2 ILGA provides a number of useful visual and textual resources on their website: https://ilga.org/
3 Remains part of the Realm of New Zealand but with significant self-determination.
4 See Aengus Carroll and Lucas Ramon Mendos, *State Sponsored Homophobia Report*, (International Lesbian, Gay, Bisexual, Trans and Intersex Association), 12th ed, 2017.
5 SBS, 'Move to Iceland: Fiji PM's advice for gay couples', (www.sbs.com.au/topics/sexuality/article/2016/01/07/move-iceland-fiji-pms-advice-gay-couples).
6 Other prominent examples of such categories are the Native American *berdache* and the Indonesian *waria*.
7 Although, as Joanna Schmidt (2010) has pointed out, such incorporation is explicitly resisted by most *fa'afafine* and Samoan culture more broadly.
8 One recent and much-reported example was the killing of a self-identified gay man by a family member in Alotau, Milne Bay in 2016. www.abc.net.au/news/2016-10-18/png-gay-community-mourns-man-allegedly-killed-by-relative/7941300.

References

Alexeyeff, K. (2008). Globalizing drag in the Cook Islands: Friction, repulsion and abjection. *The Contemporary Pacific*, 20(1), 143–161.

Altman, D. (1997). Global gaze/global gays. *GLQ: A Journal of Lesbian and Gay Studies*, 3(4), 417–436.

Altman, D. (2001). Rupture or continuity? The internationalization of gay identities. In J. C. Hawley (ed.), *Post-colonial queer: Theoretical intersections* (pp. 19–42). Albany, NY: State University of New York Press.

Besnier, Niko. 1994. Polynesian gender liminality through time and space. In G. Herdt (ed.) *Third gender: Beyond sexual dimorphism in culture and history* (pp. 285–328). New York: Zone.

Chauncey, George. (1995). *Gay New York: Gender, urban culture, and the making of the gay male world, 1890–1940*. New York: Basic Books.

Ernst, T. M. (1991). Onabasulu male homosexuality: Cosmology, affect, and prescribed male homosexuality activity among the Onabasulu of the Great Papuan Plateau. *Oceania, 62*(1), 1–11.

Herdt, G. H. (1981). *Guardians of the flutes: Idioms of masculinity*. New York: McGraw-Hill.

Herdt, G. H. (1984). Ritualized homosexual behavior: An introduction. In G. H. Herdt (Ed.), *Ritualized homosexuality in Melanesia* (pp. 1–81). Berkeley, CA: University of California Press.

Knauft, B. M. (2003). What ever happened to ritualized homosexuality? Modern sexual subjects in Melanesia and elsewhere. *Annual Review of Sex Research, 14*(1), 137–159.

Mead, M. (1928). *Coming of age in Samoa: A psychological study of primitive youth for western civilisation.* New York: William Morrow & Co.

Presterudstuen, G. H. (2014). Men trapped in women's clothing: Homosexuality, cross-dressing and manhood in Fiji. In N. Besnier and K. Alexeyeff (eds.), *Gender on the edge: Transgender, gay and other Pacific Islanders* (pp. 162–183). Honolulu, HI: University of Hawaii Press.

Presterudstuen, G. H. (2019). *Performing masculinity: Body, self, and identity in modern Fiji*. London/New York: Bloomsbury.

Schmidt, J. (2010). *Migrating genders: Westernisation, migration, and Samoan fa'afafine*. Surrey, United Kingdom: Ashgate.

Suggested further readings

Besnier, N. and K. Alexeyeff (eds). 2014. *Gender on the edge: Transgender, Gay and other Pacific Islanders*. Honolulu, HI: University of Hawaii Press.

LGBT Rights in Oceania by Equaldex: www.equaldex.com/directory/regions/oceania

International Lesbian, Gay, Bisexual, Trans and Intersex Association: https://ilga.org/.

Equaldex is a collaborative knowledge base crowdsourcing LGBT (lesbian, gay, bisexual, transgender) rights by country and region.

16

FAMILY AND DOMESTIC VIOLENCE

Yvonne Crichton-Hill and Rebecca Olul

Key points

- Family and domestic violence is costly to the Pacific in both social and economic terms.
- Key theories informing social work practice in family and domestic violence did not originate in the Pacific.
- The context within which violence occurs will influence solutions.
- Tensions exist between Pacific and Western cultural contexts and cultural perspectives.
- Responses to family and domestic violence in the Pacific should acknowledge protective factors in Pacific culture and integrate traditional and formal approaches.

Introduction

Family and domestic violence is prevalent in every society and the impacts on society can be far reaching. This chapter investigates violence in families in the Pacific region, with a special focus on Vanuatu. For the purposes of this chapter, family and domestic violence refers to any violence that occurs between family members. Even though the chapter concentrates on child abuse and neglect, and intimate partner violence, the content would have relevance for other forms of family and domestic violence.

Family and domestic violence in the Pacific region

There is limited population data in terms of family and domestic violence across the Pacific (Dunne et al., 2015; Fulu et al., 2017). While it is difficult to identify the prevalence of violence against children across the Pacific, some literature posits that violence against children is common (Dunne et al, 2015). What is certain is that violence against children results in significant harm to children and society. There are likely to be long term economic costs to society and these costs are likely to be substantial for the Pacific region if employing a burden of disease approach. The global burden of disease approach measures good health lost by using a time measure of the years of life lost to premature mortality, and the number of years lived with less than optimal health (World Health Organisation, 2017). Other literature has posited that the economic cost of child maltreatment in the Asia Pacific region ranges from $192 billion to $206 billion (Fang et al., 2015).

Across the Pacific, the speed of change economically, socially, culturally and politically varies considerably (Shek, 2017). Additionally, there exist disparities between *developed* nations and *developing* nations, such as those in the Pacific. One of the areas where disparities are evident is in relation to gender. Women in Pacific nations are underrepresented in leadership positions and therefore in decision making processes. It has been argued that this disparity can lead to a devaluing of women and children and ultimately to increased rates of domestic violence (Taylor, 2016). In terms of violence against women in the Pacific region, the literature suggests that approximately 50% of women in the Solomon Islands, Vanuatu and Fiji report experiencing some form of violence in their relationships (Taylor, 2016). The United Nations Children's Fund (UNICEF, 2014) reported that violence between partners is high across the Pacific and that there is a strong correlation between child experiences of violence and violence against women in intimate relationships. At least 78% of adults surveyed in a child protection baseline study reported physically hurting children in their household (UNICEF Pacific & Vanuatu Government, 2008). In Fiji, at least 66% of women experience some form of violence from their partner (United Nations Population Fund, 2008), while statistics for the Solomon Islands show equally high rates of violence with 64% of women having experienced violence from their intimate partner (World Health Organisation, 2013).

Key theories informing practice in family and domestic violence

Most popular in terms of understanding causes of child abuse is the work of Belsky (1993), which brings together psychological and sociological theories in an ecological framework. This work has been later developed (Keddel & Katz, 2017) where the child is placed at the centre of outwardly radiating layers of the microsystem (parents and siblings), mesosystem (school, friends, extended family), exosystem (communities, media, child welfare system) and the macrosystem (legislation culture, socio-history and economics). Social work responses to child abuse have, in the main, worked with this explanation by providing responses at various levels of the ecological framework, from programmes involving work with parents through to attitude and behaviour change programmes to educate communities and society about the harm that can be caused by child abuse and neglect. Ultimately, theories about child abuse and neglect

> embody beliefs about what child rearing behaviour is unacceptable or dangerous and values about people: the relative rights of adults and children, the relative value of males and females. Hence, there is considerable variation over time and between cultures in what is deemed abusive.
> (Munro, 2002, p. 50)

In terms of violence against women, the most influential theory to explain its occurrence in the Western world is feminist theory. Feminist analysis developed from an understanding that, overwhelmingly, violence in intimate adult relationships is carried out by men towards women. Feminist theory suggested that this reflects a patriarchal societal structure aimed at subordinating women (McPhail et al., 2007) and which is maintained through the process of socialisation where children are taught traditional male and female roles where "femininity is strongly associated with conquest and masculinity with domination" (Cribb, 1999, p. 51). The feminist movement has influenced the development of individual empowerment work with women and children through the provision of education programmes, safe houses and refuges. However, more recently, in some parts of the world, there has been a move towards a more holistic and family centred approach to working with violence against women.

Definitions and theories about family and domestic violence are culturally bound, as are the responses communities and societies develop to counter violence. One example of culturally contextualised theorising about domestic and family violence is Nga Vaka o Kainga Tapu (Ministry of Social Development, 2012). This series of eight ethnic specific frameworks was developed by Pacific communities, professionals and spiritual leaders in New Zealand. The frameworks derive from Pacific values, beliefs and theorising, and are intended to inform policy and practice responses to violence.

Reflection question

How can theories that have originated elsewhere be applied to family and domestic violence in Pacific nations?

Contextualising violence in the Pacific

The occurrence of violence in the Pacific is influenced by a number of factors including: unequal gender and power relations (Government of Vanuatu & UNICEF, 2005); a belief that violence is part of traditional culture (Australian Government, 2014); a perception that violence is a family affair and not for the wider community (Fairbairn-Dunlop, 2009); traditional or "*kastom*" marriage practices, such as the bride price, that are perceived to give license to men to abuse their wives; and, economic reasons inhibiting women from leaving violent relationships (Government of Vanuatu & UNICEF, 2005). Furthermore, there are a range of tensions that might exist between Pacific and Western cultural contexts and cultural perspectives. Next, these tensions are explored.

Collective/communal versus individual contexts

Pacific cultures have been described as collective or communal cultures. Primarily, this means that Pacific cultures are strongly relational and gain a sense of belonging and strength of identity from belonging to a Pacific community (Crichton-Hill, 2017; Ministry of Social Development, 2012). In cultures that value the collective, there is often a shared responsibility for health and well-being (Ihara & Vakalahi, 2012). Conversely, responses to family and domestic violence have been individualistic in nature emanating from a feminist and criminal justice approach where the perpetrator of the violence faces individual consequences and where social work practice is intent on protecting individual women and children from violence.

Traditional (customary law) versus legal responses

It has been suggested that legal approaches to family and domestic violence are not well utilised with very few Pacific nations possessing targeted civil and criminal domestic violence legislation (Forster, 2011). There is a danger that legislative responses reflect the values of the colonising powers rather than the indigenous population for whom the legislative response is devised. In terms of traditional approaches, Forster (2011) further argued that traditional reconciliation processes in the Pacific may be conducted without the consent of female victims of violence. In fact, sometimes family and domestic violence can be supported by traditional and religious leaders (Pacific Women, 2017).

The data from studies into family and domestic violence in the Pacific has been used to advocate for legislative changes, with Vanuatu being one of the first to introduce legislation specific to family violence in 2009. For example, the Family Protection Act criminalises domestic violence and provides for protection orders for up to two years for the protection of victims of family violence (VWC & VNSO, 2011; UN Women, 2010). Temporary protection orders may be granted by Authorised Persons in areas where there are no courts for up to 14 days with possibility for extension for a further 14 days. The Act also protects children from family violence (VWC & VNSO, 2011; UN Women, 2010).

In the Solomon Islands, the Family Protection Bill was passed by parliament in late 2014. It was the first of its kind, creating a legal framework that deals with domestic violence as a criminal offence. The Act provides protection for all family members from all forms of violence.

For nations that have introduced family and domestic violence legislation, the challenge now lies in implementing and enforcing that law, and in creating an environment that encourages and enables women to have access to the formal justice system, as well as effective survivor services.

Informal systems versus formal systems

It is understood that many women in violent relationships will first turn to informal systems of family and friends before seeking assistance from more formal networks such as the police or organisations working in the violence field. The literature reports that a woman's relationships with her family and friends can be impacted, especially if there have been threats to family safety by the perpetrator, at which point families may attempt to distance themselves (Latta & Goodman, 2011). A challenge exists when there are limited formal systems available and when informal systems are not supportive of those who have experienced family and domestic violence, leaving women and children with limited opportunities for help seeking. In fact, most women in Pacific nations do not report family and domestic violence due to threats, fear of reprisal and a lack of confidence in formal and informal services (Pacific Women, 2017).

Rural settings versus urban settings

Rural social work literature contends that social workers in rural areas will face challenges in engaging resources and specialised services (Parrish & Trawver, 2013). In Pacific nations, geographic isolation and lack of a transport infrastructure, along with cultural norms supporting violence, is likely to impact the reporting of family and domestic violence (Pacific Women, 2017). Similarly, there are likely to be challenges facing social workers who work with family violence in urban areas, especially where there is an under resourcing of services to provide support to families who experience violence. The following two case studies highlight the contextual issues facing social work in urban and rural settings in the Pacific Island nation of Vanuatu.

CASE STUDY 16.1: FAMILY AND DOMESTIC VIOLENCE IN URBAN VANUATU

Marie, a 21 year old woman, lives in Vanuatu, a small island developing state in the Pacific Ocean with a population of 272,500 (VNSO, 2009).

Unemployed and a victim of violence at the hands of her husband, Marie resides in Port Vila, with her husband and two children under the age of seven. Marie's husband is the sole breadwinner in the family. He often hits the children as well. The most comprehensive study on family violence and intimate partner violence[1] in Vanuatu shows alarmingly high rates of violence against women by husbands/partners: among women who have ever been married, lived with a man, or had an intimate sexual relationship with a partner, three in five experienced physical and/or sexual violence in their lifetime (VWC & VNSO, 2011). Marie is part of the alarming statistics. She fears not just for herself but also for her children.

Options available to women like Marie include: police and the judicial system; traditional or "*kastom*" law administered by chiefs; mediation by religious leaders; and women's crisis centres.[2]

Marie's sister informed her of the Family Protection Unit of the Vanuatu Police Force that deals primarily with rape cases[3] but also with domestic violence cases. Marie went to the Family Protection Unit for support, where she was referred to the Vanuatu Women's Centre for counselling. A legal officer helped Marie apply for a temporary protection order. The Vanuatu Women's Centre, one of the only providers of survivor services, provides advocacy, legal services and education on family violence.

Activity questions

What are the key issues presented in the case study that social workers working in urban Vanuatu should pay attention to?
What steps might you take to address these issues?

CASE STUDY 16.2: FAMILY AND DOMESTIC VIOLENCE IN RURAL VANUATU

Matan, a mother of four in her late 30s, lives in a rural village in east Pentecost. At least 80% of Vanuatu's population reside in rural and remote villages scattered throughout the widespread islands, like Matan. The geographic spread, high costs related to accessing services and socio-cultural challenges mean many difficulties face women like Matan accessing support services.

Matan's husband of over 10 years is a well-respected leader in the community. The community knows that he hits Matan.

With high rates of violence against women by husbands/partners, there is a need to strengthen services in rural Vanuatu to respond to violence and sexual abuse (VWC & VNSO, 2011). Access to justice is limited in rural remote Vanuatu where the bulk of the population lives and where there are high rates of intimate partner violence (VWC & VNSO, 2011). In remote locations, police presence is limited to nonexistent. Matan will need to travel a great distance (up to five hours of walking) or travel quicker but at an exorbitant cost (up to USD400 on a seven-metre fiberglass outboard motor boat in open sea), placing herself at great risk of harm of further violence from her husband should he become aware of her actions to seek support.

Additionally, Matan does not agree with her husband hitting the older two children. She mentioned this to the chief in the community.

Traditional justice exists within the "*kastom*" law and chiefly systems and is more widely available for women and children in rural Vanuatu with a goal of preserving family harmony over individual justice. Women report being disadvantaged within this system due to chiefs being male and hearings occurring in the community "*nakamal*", a place women have no access to and do not have a voice (Fairbairn-Dunlop, 2009; UN Women, 2010).

At an education session in her community, Matan learned about the role of Vanuatu Women's Centre and its Committee against Violence against Women. She reached out to a committee representative in her village for advice and support.

Activity questions

How might responses to rural Vanuatu be strengthened?
What knowledge, resources or skills would you need to implement service strengthening plans to rural Vanuatu?

Practice approaches

As is highlighted by the contrasting tensions in the previous section, there is a danger of intellectual colonisation (Ravulo, 2016) where external social work frameworks are given priority, thereby undervaluing indigenous frameworks which have grown out of the context in which violence is embedded. Sometimes, to incorporate cultural perspectives, social workers might make surface amendments to material or publications used in work with families. An example is the translating of information into other languages. While this might seem like a useful idea, the alterations do nothing to embed the cultural values of the target population into the content provided to families (Reece, Vera & Caldwell, 2006) and is therefore an example of professional colonisation.

Social work practice in Pacific nations must be grounded in the values and practices of Pacific cultures. After all, violence is contextually located and context will influence solutions. Therefore, social work in the Pacific in the area of family and domestic violence must be cognisant of the contextual realities of social disadvantage, poverty and discrimination which exist throughout much of the Pacific region. As noted earlier, a range of issues including acceptance of violence, tolerance of gender inequality, social inequality, limited services to support children, women and families, poverty and a lack of policies and programmes to deal with violence increase the likelihood that domestic and family violence will occur (WHO & ISPCAN, 2006). In addition, "South Pacific nations face various development challenges, including climate change, health, education and infrastructure development" (Mafile'o & Vakalahi, 2016, p. 3). These factors must be considered in any practice approach to the issue.

For these reasons, responses to family and domestic violence in the Pacific must be multidimensional and address micro and macro factors and respond to family and community systems holistically. In other words, responses should include prevention efforts alongside crisis intervention, work with individuals, families and communities, work with women, men and children, and policy and legislative change. Social work, with its focus on building relationships, enhancing wellbeing, promoting social change and working with indigenous populations (see International Federation of Social Workers definition of social work: http://ifsw.org/) should be well placed to respond to family and domestic violence in Pacific nations. Complementary to family and domestic violence, social work in the Pacific is the acknowledgement of culture as a protective factor and a focus on integrating traditional and formal approaches.

Harnessing culture as a protective factor

There are social and cultural norms, and cultural factors, such as those highlighted earlier, that promote protective factors central to violence prevention and intervention. Protective factors can promote resilience in three areas: in terms of mitigating the likelihood that violence will occur; promoting resilience post violence; and mediating the impact of violence. In the Pacific, collectively based community structures and networks, shared caring of children within extended families, some traditional responses to cultural transgressions, and community based initiatives led by non-government organisations, Governments and institutions such as UNICEF can be noted as protective and resilience building. For example, in Vanuatu UNICEF is supporting the Ministry of Justice and Community Services and relevant protection agencies to pilot in identified communities a child protection community facilitation package that builds on and strengthens existing community mechanisms for the protection of children. This is to complement the Government's Family and Traditional Child Protection System model and address research findings that police divert at least 95% of the cases they deal with to the community (UNICEF Pacific & Vanuatu Government, 2008). Highlighted is the need to focus on traditional and community actors to ensure they are fully engaged in child protection. The community facilitation package targets parents, caregivers, chiefs, community and faith based leaders and youth leaders, and builds on the traditional ways children are valued and cherished that likens nurturing of children to raising yams (UNICEF Pacific, 2016), a highly valued crop used for custom ceremonies throughout many islands in Vanuatu. To this end, community child protection volunteers have been nominated and a community child protection body set up that has responsibilities for carrying out and monitoring a community action plan (UNICEF Pacific, 2016).

A burgeoning body of research has highlighted the relationship between cultural identity, cultural engagement and violence, stating that cultural engagement contributes to violence desistance (Austin, 2004; Irwin et al., 2017). So how might culture be embedded in violence work in the Pacific? As an example, in mitigating the likelihood that violence will occur (violence prevention), Pacific cultural values and norms can mediate changes in attitudes and behaviours. For prevention, social work to be culturally meaningful to the Pacific population, the following must be considered:

The particular Pacific community's

- Natural or traditional prevention strategies
- Methods of organising information
- Means of communicating information

Including the Pacific community and especially prevention participants in the planning, implementation and evaluation of prevention efforts is one way of confirming Pacific cultural norms and beliefs are embedded in the work being done.

Integrating traditional and formal approaches

Different cultural communities will employ different processes to achieve healing and restoration. An example of the integration of traditional (customary) and formal approaches is evidenced through the role of the Women's Centre in Vanuatu.

In Vanuatu, the main service provider of counselling services to victims of family violence, awareness raising, legal aid and advocacy on family violence is the non-governmental organisation Vanuatu Women's Centre. Due to the geographic spread of the country, Vanuatu Women's Centre has provincial arms in at least four of the provinces and has set up a network called Committee against Violence against Women (CAVAW). At least 37 active island-based CAVAWs work throughout all the 6 provinces of Vanuatu to undertake community awareness at the local level and support women and children living in violence in remote communities. CAVAWs work together with male advocates that include chiefs, pastors, police, health workers and youth leaders that the Vanuatu Women's Centre trains to advocate on the elimination of violence (VWC & VNSO, 2011). This helps to ensure that the protective mechanisms already in place at the community level are drawn on and strengthened to provide protection of families from violence.

Conclusion

We conclude this chapter as we started it, with the recognition that family and domestic violence is prevalent across many societies. Family and domestic violence in Pacific nations presents social work with a number of unique challenges. A comprehensive social work response that takes account of these challenges, and the cultural context from which the challenges arise, is needed to protect Pacific women and children and to enhance family and community wellbeing.

Notes

1 Women's Centre (VWC) and the Vanuatu National Statistics Office (VNSO), (2011).
2 Government of Vanuatu & UNICEF, 2005.
3 UN Women, 2010.

References

Austin, A. A. (2004). Alcohol, tobacco, other drug use, and violent behavior among Native Hawaiians: Ethnic pride and resilience. *Substance Use & Misuse, 39*(5), 721–746. doi: 10.1081/JA-120034013

Australian Government. (2014). *Pacific women shaping Pacific development. Design document.* Australia: Department of Foreign Affairs and Trade.

Belsky, J. (1993). Etiology of child maltreatment: A developmental-ecological analysis. *Psychological Bulletin, 114*(3), 413–434. 10.1037/0033-2909.114.3.413

Cribb, J. O. (1999). Being bashed: Western Samoan women's responses to domestic violence in Western Samoa and New Zealand. *Gender, Place & Culture, 6*(1), 49–65. doi: 10.1080/09663699925141

Crichton-Hill, Y. I. (2017). Pasifika social work. In M. Connolly, L. Harms & J. Maidment (Eds.), *Social work contexts and practice* (4th ed.): 109–120. Sydney, Australia: Oxford University Press.

Dunne, M. P., Choo, W. Y., Madrid, B., Subrahmanian, R., Rumble, L., Blight, S. & Maternowska, M. C. (2015). Violence against children in the Asia Pacific Region: The situation is becoming clearer. *Asia Pacific Journal of Public Health, 27*(8), 6S–8S. doi: 10.1177/1010539515602184

Fairbairn-Dunlop, P. (2009). *Pacific prevention of domestic violence programme: Vanuatu report.* Wellington: Pacific Police Prevention of Domestic Violence & NZ Aid.

Fang, X., Fry, D., Brown, D., Mercy, J. A, Dunne, M. P., Butchart, A. R. ... Swales, D. M. (2015). The burden of child maltreatment in the East Asia and Pacific Region. *Child Abuse & Neglect, 42*, 146–162.

Forster, C. (2011). Ending domestic violence in Pacific Island countries: The critical role of law. *Asian-Pacific Law & Policy Journal, 12*(2), 123–144.

Fulu, E., Miedema, S., Roselli, T., McCook, S., Chan, K. L., Haardörfer, R. & Jewkes, R. (2017). Pathways between childhood trauma, intimate partner violence, and harsh parenting: Findings from the UN multi-country study on men and violence in Asia and the Pacific. *The Lancet Global Health, 5*(5), e512–e522. doi.org/10.1016/S2214-109X(17)30103-1

Government of Vanuatu & UNICEF. (2005). *Vanuatu, a situation analysis of children, women and youth.* Fiji: UNICEF Pacific Office.

Ihara, E. S. & Vakalahi, H. F. O. (2012). Collective worldviews and health of Pacific American elders. *Educational Gerontology*, *38*(6), 400–411. doi:10.1080/03601277.2011.559852

Irwin, K., Mossakowski, K., Spencer, J. H., Umemoto, K. N., Hishinuma, E. S., Garcia-Santiago, O. … Choi-Misailidis, S. (2017). Do different dimensions of ethnic identity reduce the risk of violence among Asian American and Pacific Islander adolescents in Hawai'i? *Journal of Human Behavior in the Social Environment*, *27*(3), 151–164. doi: 10.1080/10911359.2016.1262806

Keddell, E. & Katz, I. (2017). Working in child and family welfare. In M. Connolly, L. Harms & J. Maidment (Eds.), *Social work contexts and practice*. (4th ed.). Sydney, Australia: Oxford University Press.

Latta, R. E. & Goodman, L. A. (2011). Intervening in partner violence against women: A grounded theory exploration of informal network members' experiences. *The Counseling Psychologist*, *39*(7), 973–1023. doi: 10.1177/0011000011398504

Mafile'o, T. & Vakalahi, H. F. O. (2016). Indigenous social work across borders: Expanding social work in the South Pacific. *International Social Work*, *61*(4). doi: 10.1177/0020872816641750

McPhail, B. A., Busch, N. B., Kulkarni, S. & Rice, G. (2007). An integrative feminist model: The evolving feminist perspective on intimate partner violence. *Violence Against Women*, *13*(8), 817–841. doi: 10.1177/1077801207302039

Ministry of Social Development. (2012). *Nga vaka o kaiga tapu. A Pacific conceptual framework to address family violence in New Zealand*. Wellington, New Zealand: Ministry of Social Development.

Munro, E. P. (2002). *Effective child protection*. London: SAGE Publications.

Pacific Women. (2017). *Ending violence against women. Roadmap Synthesis Report. Informing the Pacific women shaping Pacific development roadmap 2017–2022*. Australia: Australian Aid.

Parrish, D. E. & Trawver, K. R. (2013). Evidence-based practice in the rural context. In T. L. Scales, C. L. Streeter & H. S. Cooper (Eds.), *Rural social work: Building and sustaining community capacity* (pp. 131–143). Hoboken, NJ: John Wiley & Sons Incorporated.

Ravulo, J. (2016). Pacific epistemologies in professional social work practice, policy and research. *Asia Pacific Journal of Social Work and Development*, *26*(4), 191–202. doi: 10.1080/02185385.2016.1234970

Reese, L. E., Vera, E. M. & Caldwell, L. D. (2006). The role and function of culture in violence prevention practice and science. In J. Lutzker, R. (Ed.), *Preventing violence: Research and evidence-based intervention strategies* (pp. 259–278). Washington, DC: American Psychological Association.

Shek, D. T. L. (2017). Editorial: A snapshot of social work in the Asia-Pacific region. *The British Journal of Social Work*, *47*(1), 1–8. https://doi.org/10.1093/bjsw/bcx007

Taylor, C. (2016). Domestic violence and its prevalence in small island developing states – South Pacific region. *Pacific Journal of Reproductive Health*, *1*(3), 119–127.

UN Women. (2010). *Ending violence against women & girls. Evidence, data and knowledge in the Pacific Island Countries. Literature review and annotated bibliography*. Geneva, Switzerland: United Nations.

UNICEF Pacific. (2016). Vanuatu update, July–August 2016. www.unicef.org/pacificislands/UNICEF_Pacific_in_Vanuatu_Jul-Aug_2016_Partner_Update.pdf

United Nations Children's Fund. (2014). *Violence against children in East Asia and the Pacific: A regional review and synthesis of findings, strengthening child protection series, No. 4*. Bangkok, Thailand: UNICEF EAPRO.

United Nations Children's Fund & the Vanuatu Government. (2008). *Protect me with love and care. A baseline report for creating a future free from violence, abuse and exploitation of girls and boys in Vanuatu*. Fiji: UNICEF Pacific Sub Regional Office.

United Nations Population Fund. (2008). *An assessment of the state of violence against women*. Fiji: United Nations Population Fund Pacific Sub Regional Office.

Vanuatu National Statistics Office, Government of Vanuatu. (2009). *2009 National Population and Housing Census*. Port Vila, Vanuatu: Government of Vanuatu.

Vanuatu Women's Centre in partnership with the Vanuatu National Statistics Office. (2011). *Vanuatu National Survey on Women's Lives and Family Relationships*. Port Vila, Vanuatu.

World Health Organisation. (2013). *Social Determinants of Health. Country Case: Violence against women in Solomon Islands. Translating research into policy and action on the social determinants of health*. Manila: World Health Organisation Office for the Western Pacific Region.

World Health Organisation. (2017). *WHO methods and data sources for global burden of disease estimates 2000–2015*. Geneva, Switzerland: World Health Organisation.

Suggested further readings/websites

Australian Aid. Pacific Women Shaping Pacific Development:
https://pacificwomen.org/our-work/focus-areas/ending-violence-against-women/
www.pasefikaproud.co.nz/resources/

17

GLOBAL MIGRATION AND RESETTLEMENT

A case study on the Fijian experience

Litea Meo-Sewabu

Key points

- Fijians have moved across the Oceania region and beyond, and settled within these new areas with a view to utilise both indigenous perspective alongside contemporary local perspectives.
- The need to connect with Vanua, or the land, is part of this bigger process that enable Fijians to still practice and implement traditional views across their new localities.
- Ensuring indigenous perspectives are meaningfully included in the many facets of policy will ensure wellbeing is upheld and protected for the Pacific diaspora.

Fijian migration across the Oceania region

Historically, Pacific peoples have always navigated Oceania to exchange goods, trade and provide services. In doing so, these exchanges have brought a heightened awareness of key relationships and in essence have strengthened and maintained relationships across Oceania and worldwide. These exchanges now occur globally through skilled migration, sports and government work schemes including seasonal work within the agriculture sector. Remittances earned by migrant workers contributes to the livelihood of families living in the islands and builds transnational migrant communities all across Oceania. This chapter focuses on migration to Aotearoa (New Zealand) and Australia and discusses issues of transnational identities and how cultural capital is maintained.

Since the 2006 census, Pacific peoples in Aotearoa have increased from 6.9% (265,974) to 7.4% (295,941) of the total population of 4,608,796, of which 14,445 are Fijians (Statistics New Zealand, 2014). The statistics indicate that the Fijian population in Aotearoa had increased by 40% since the census in 2001, the highest amongst all of the Pacific population groups.

Fijians, along with the Pacific population, migrated to Aotearoa in the early 1970s as Aotearoa offered work schemes to most Pacific countries in order to address manual labour shortages (Krishnan, Schoeffel & Warren, 1994). Most Fijians were recruited into the agriculture and forestry industry in Takoroa, Hawkes Bay, Whanganui and Waikato (Vunidilo, 2008). Fijians still remain in these regions, but a large population group have settled in Whanganui. Canterbury also has a significant population of Fijians who migrated to work within their forest industries and still remain there to this day. In the 1980s and 1990s, there have been a stream of Telecom (a local telecommunications company now called Spark in Aotearoa) workers and skilled workers from Fiji migrating into Aotearoa. The numerous military *coup d'état* in Fiji has also increased the migration of highly skilled workers into Aotearoa and other parts of the world, now referred to as the "brain drain", meaning the migration of well-educated citizens from Fiji (Vunidilo, 2008).

Fijian identity and the transnational community

Vertovec (2009) views transnational communities as a phenomenon that brings people together based on a shared culture, religious beliefs or geographical origin. Within the Aotearoa context, Spoonley (2001) explains transnationalism within a Pacific community as communities who have links between their current place of residence and their place of origin. He adds that these communities strategically use resources in both places and social and cultural capital exchanges as necessary for the maintenance of kinships and relationships through which Pacific identities are crafted. In terms of how culture and Indigenous knowledge is maintained, Durie (2004) states that:

> while indigenous knowledge is often valued because of its traditional qualities, a creative and inventive capacity forms the core of indigenous knowledge systems ... , arising from the creative potential of indigenous knowledge is the prospect that it can be applied to modern times in parallel with other knowledge systems.
>
> *(p. 1139)*

Durie's statement emphasises that Indigenous knowledge can be applied in transnational communities and in modern times, the forms of transmitting the culture may vary, giving rise to a new body of knowledge within these transient communities.

Hence, it is important to note that reference to the notion of "community" in this chapter refers to the reconstructed community participants now call home.

This reconstructed community is a space that they have become a part of, outside of Fiji; and intuitively have set out to participate in this community in order to maintain their cultural identity as Indigenous Fijians. Vertovec (2009) describes the common cultural linkages that bring a group or society together as transnationalism, defined as:

> sustained linkages and on-going exchanges among non-state actors based across national borders-businesses, non-governmental organizations, and individuals sharing the same interest by way of criteria such as religion beliefs, common cultural and geographic origins practices and … these[are] transnational practices … their links functioning across nation-states.
>
> *(p. 3)*

Fijian communities like many Indigenous groups are connected by their sense of belonging to the *Vanua* or the land. The *Vanua* forms part of a reconstructed community because it is a space that has been recreated with varying forms of the Fijian culture and tradition. These cultural forms are influenced by transnational forces within a transnational community. These influences can be in the form of information flows through forms of technology, social media and institutions as well as other social forces that can shape and influence worldviews and perspectives. The communal space allows its citizens to maintain their cultural identity as Indigenous Fijians. Cultural identity is then based on relationships within the *Vanua*. Social, cultural and capital exchanges occur globally to maintain connection with the *Vanua* and the collective culture. This flow of exchanges has been likened to a form of "transnational cooperation", and is also referred to as transnationalism (Hulkenberg, 2015). Within Oceanic cultures, these exchanges, despite living in diaspora, allows us to maintain our sense of belonging to the *Vanua*.

Communal wellbeing in the example of the *solesolevaki* relates to the concept of social capital. Social capital was first defined by Putnam (2000) as "the collective value of all social networks and the inclination that arise from these networks to do things for each other" (p. 135). It is further elaborated as "features of social organisation, such as trust, norms and networks that can improve the efficiency of society by facilitating coordinated actions" (Putnam, Leonardi, and Nanetti 1993, p. 167). These definitions continue to evolve, but all focus on the importance of building a communal cohesiveness, hence a sense of communal wellbeing. Veenstra and Patterson (2012) note that "relatively few studies have addressed the interconnectedness of social capital with institutionalised cultural and economic capital as determinants of health" (p. 280).

PRACTICE EXAMPLE 17.1

Reciprocity and gift giving is an integral part of Fijian culture and collective cultures. A story was once relayed to me about a man from Oceania residing in Aotearoa, who for years had continuously given to his community. His daughter was to be married and he was on his way to the bank to get a loan for his daughter's wedding when members of the community came for a visit. They had an envelope that contained the community's collection to assist with the wedding. There was no need for him to get a loan as the collection was well over what he needed. All over Oceania, reciprocity is the essence of our communal and collective value that capitalises on social capital and is not time specific. We do this for weddings, for funerals, for birthdays and for births, in the village and wherever we live globally. This example is a classic case of communal wellbeing and even in Aotearoa gift giving is important and keeps them connected to the traditions of the Vanua.

As Pacific communities have become a part of the diaspora, they continue to bring their communities together using the concepts of "*solesolevaki*" in events such as weddings, funerals and birthdays. The relationships are formed because of their connection to Oceania. It is this sense of connection that draws transnational communities together to support one another. Through *solesolevaki* they will work together to prepare for the event and contribute either in cash or in kind by bringing whatever is needed to make the event complete and a success. Nothing is expected in return because of the concept of reciprocity – it is believed that a favour will be returned when needed, it is not time specific but is bound to occur at some point.

Transnationalism and the Vanua

Identity is not confined to a narrow geographical space as in the Island village, however, attributes of wellbeing identified from the village such as 1) *Dau veiqaravi* (to be of service), 2) *Taucoko ni qaravi itavi* (completion and completeness of tasks), 3) *Na veiwekani* (maintaining harmony), 4) *Ke nai i rairai* (physical appearance) and 5) *Bula vakayalo* (spirituality) are visible or also practiced in Aotearoa within Fijian communal gatherings. The forms in which these practices are displayed differed as they have become part of transnational community. The core value though remain the same but practiced is various forms within the transnational communities they have become a part of.

The first criteria, "*Dau veiqaravi*" or to be of service, was more visible in communal gatherings with members of the Fijian community in the area and in some instances this value extended to other ethnic groups within their local neighbourhood. The second criteria, "*Taucoko ni qaravi itavi*" or completion and completeness of tasks, was also visible in their participation in *Vanua* social structures in Aotearoa, Fiji and globally. Engagement with *Vanua* social structures as well as local institutions enable Fijians to participate in their community regardless of geographical space. Cultivating relationships within these global communities were seen as contributing to overall wellbeing through maintaining their cultural identity. The third criteria of maintaining harmony is carried out using modern technology and other forms to maintain the kinships regardless which part of the world they reside. Fijians also identified a fourth criterion on physical appearance as in Fiji, participants focused on physical appearance as a source of wellbeing. In Aotearoa, the focus incorporates and shifts to an emphasis on physical activity. Being physically active through gardening and going for a walk to visit friends were all seen as forms of exercise. Overall, Fijians also stressed the importance of the fifth criteria, spirituality.

Integrating Fijian perspective into policy

In defining the health of Indigenous peoples, the United Nations Permanent Forum on Indigenous Issues (2009) stated that the concept of health "is shaped by Indigenous peoples" (p. 157) historical experiences and worldviews, and is expressed in the rules and norms that are applied in the community and practised by its members. In Aotearoa, Fijian's cultural identity as Indigenous Fijians remained an integral part of their lives and determined how they perceived themselves in the reconstructed community.

There are varying definitions of social policy in Aotearoa/New Zealand (Cheyne, O'Brien & Belgrave, 2008) and globally (Spicker, 2014) although in general all definitions highlight a course of action taken to bring about positive outcomes. The author acknowledges that there is an inherent tension within policy analysis as social policies have uneven impacts on different groups within a population, making it highly unlikely that all people in a society will benefit from any particular policy initiative.

The concern for most Indigenous populations, however, is that social policies often utilise western paradigms without due consideration of their effectiveness in addressing issues facing Indigenous peoples who are often the targets of social policies. There is an increasing recognition primarily from within Indigenous communities that Indigenous voices should be heard within social policy, which means that traditional meanings, words and ways of knowing all need to be reflected within the social policies of their countries (Durie, 2005; Hokowhitu, 2010).

Wellbeing is defined from a Fijian perspective and the various contexts, in which contemporary understandings of wellbeing are embedded, can be summarised as follows. Nabobo-Baba (2006) refers to wellbeing as "*sautu*" or the good quality of life that enables the *Vanua* or people to be healthy and wealthy (p. 155). *Sautu* or *bula taucoko* in relation to social policy can also be achieved by examining policies that protect those who are most vulnerable within the *Vanua*; these policies are referred to as social protection policies. Social protection, according to Rotuivaqali (2012, p. 4) has been used interchangeably in the Pacific with terms such as, "social security, social insurance, social pensions and social safety nets ... social protection is what a society collectively does to protect its weakest member in order to meet the social needs of all" (p. 4).

The definition of social protection as defined by Ratuva (2010) explores cultural systems that can be used in the informal systems as safety nets to protect the most vulnerable within the community. Globally, literature tells us that female headed households remain the most vulnerable economically compared to male headed households (UN Women, 2015). Similarly, in Fijian literature it indicates that women headed households remain economically disadvantaged (Pabon, Umapathi & Waqavonovono, 2012), yet policies are silent about specifying gender realities of women in Fiji.

Social policy, equality and human rights

A major tension for policy making and the wellbeing of Indigenous communities' world-wide has been the creation of appropriate social work approaches and who has the power to determine what worldviews inform such strategies. For example, the impacts of colonisation in Australia, Aotearoa, Fiji and other Pacific Island Countries (PICs) continue to influence the development of social work, at times with questionable results. There is an urgency to develop and use frameworks that are inclusive of Indigenous worldviews, and that consider localised solutions that affirm traditional social structures and cultural practices in the development of social work education, practice, policy and research.

Durie's (2005) framework for social policy alongside of Nabobo-Baba's (2006, 2008) and Baba et al.'s (2013) examination of wellbeing and the *Vanua* as well as Ratuva's (2010) explanation of social protection offers opportunities for two Indigenous cultures from Oceania to weave together their stories and to consider how social policies can and should preserve cultural heritage and wellbeing. Madraiwiwi (2008) sums up the importance of a collective approach in the case of Fiji, stating that, "unless we collectively commit ourselves to reconstructing or re-fashioning our own epistemologies, the risk is that others will define us" (p. 4). However, in Aotearoa, there has been progress as in the case of the Maori Party providing a critical Indigenous voice to political debates.

The indigenous context in promoting relevant Pacific policy in practice

When it comes to health, education, justice, housing and welfare, Maori in Aotearoa and Indigenous migrant population groups such as Pacific peoples are at the brunt of social policies which have not necessarily benefited or helped to address the social problems within their communities (Meo-Sewabu &

Walsh-Tapiata, 2012). Furthermore, countries subjected to Western colonisation often emphasise individual freedom as the foundation of modern society, while the collective nature of family villages and tribes is rarely acknowledged. Social work has therefore often been based on western philosophies and values with the expectation that Indigenous communities will change or conform to them. In addition, social policies within most developing countries continues to be driven by the Northern hemisphere governments and experts who often do not understand the cultural structures nor the daily realities of Indigenous communities (Connell, 2007).

Social policy frameworks mostly address issues relating to material deprivation, and yet Indigenous groups often have different indicators which reflect their wellbeing. Wellbeing, for example in findings from this case study, is referred to as "*bula taucoko* and *bula sautu*". Findings relating to *bula sautu* identify that a sense of belonging; valuing relationships; and completion of tasks and roles are all intangible Indigenous values that are often not incorporated into social policy goals that are based in Western conceptual frameworks.

Conclusion

Therefore, there is an urgency to develop and use frameworks that are inclusive of Indigenous world views, and that consider localised solutions that affirm traditional social structures and cultural practices in the development of social work. This includes promoting social work approaches that allow collective structures to work together. Durie (2005, 2011) suggests that unity with the natural environment, or *Vanua* (land), is the primary defining characteristic of Indigenous peoples, along with secondary characteristics that include celebrating custom and group interaction. This then gives rise to a system of knowledge, facilitating sustainable economic growth and contributing to a unique language.

REFLECTIVE QUESTIONS

1. What are some informal systems and safety nets in indigenous and transnational communities?
2. There is a belief that it is more important to assimilate to the new culture within the new country Pacific people may find themselves migrating to. How might this negatively impact on maintaining positive connections to *vanua* and overall wellbeing?
3. How can we utilise cultural terms (like those listed in the glossary in Table 17.1) more effectively when working with the Fijian diaspora?

TABLE 17.1 Glossary of terms used within Chapter

B
Bula taucoko: The achievement of a state of completion.

I
iTaukei: Indigenous Fijians as owners of the land.
itovo vakavanua: Protocols and cultural practices and processes with the Indigenous Fijian culture.

K
Kava: Common name for yaqona, a ceremonial drink.

M
Marama-iTaukei: Indigenous Fijian woman.

N
Na i tovo vakaviti: Fijian way of life, involving customs and traditions.

S
Sautu: Wellbeing or the good quality life of the *vanua* or people.
Sevusevu: Acknowledging entrance to the land or *Vanua*.
Solesolevaki: To work together to achieve a common purpose making mats, gardening.

T
Talanoa: Sharing of conversation and knowledge.
Tali magimagi: Used as a metaphor to talk about things in detail.
Tanoa: Bowl used to drink yaqona.
Tokatoka: Family units.

V
Vakamarama: A female having characteristics and qualities that bestows respect.
Vakaturaga: A male having characteristics and qualities that bestows respect; is said to be chieflike.
Vakarau vakavanua: The practices of the land or Vanua.
Vanua: The way of knowing, refers to "a people, their chief, their defined territory, their waterways or fishing grounds, their environment, their spirituality, their history, their epistemology and culture" (Nabobo-Baba, 2006, p. 155).
Vasu: Primarily defined as the village connection through the mother or the maternal links to a village.
Veikauwaitaki: Thinking of others.
Veidokai: Respect-to show respect.
Veisiko: To visit someone.
Veiwasei: Sharing with others.

Y
Yaqona: Also known as *kava* or the traditional Fijian drink.
Yavusa: Group of families populating a village.
Yalo: Spirit.
Yalomatua: Considered wise.

References

Baba, T., Boladuadua, E. L., Ba, T., Vatuloka, W. V. & Nabobo-Baba, U. (2013). *Na vuku ni vanua = Wisdom of the land: Aspects of Fijian knowledge, culture and history*. Suva, Fiji: Native Academy Publishers, Institute of Indigenous Studies, Fiji (IISF).

Cheyne, C., O'Brien, M., & Belgrave, M. (2008). *Social policy in Aotearoa New Zealand* (4th ed.). Auckland, New Zealand: Oxford University Press.

Connell, R. (2007). *Southern theory: The global dynamics of knowledge in social science*. Crows Nest, Australia: Allen & Unwin.

Durie, M. (2004). An Indigenous Model of Health Promotion. *18th World Conference on Health Promotion and Health Education*. Retrieved from http://temata.massey.ac.nz/doc/Health_Promotion_and_Health_Education.pdf

Durie, M. (2005). Race and ethnicity in public policy: Does it work? *Social Policy Journal of New Zealand, 24*, 1–11.

Durie, M. (2011). *Nga tini whetu: Navigating Maori futures*. Wellington, New Zealand: Huia Publishers.

Hokowhitu, B. (2010). A genealogy of indigenous resistance. In B. Hokowhitu, N. Kermoal, C. Anderson, M. Reilly, A. Peterson, I. Altamirano-Jimenez & P. Rewi (Eds.), *Indigenous identity and resistance: Researching the diversity of knowledge* (pp. 207–225). Dunedin, New Zealand: Otago University Press.

Hulkenberg, J. (2015). Fijian kinship: Exchange and migration. In C. Toren & S. Pauwels (eds.) *Living kinship in the Pacific*. New York: Berghahn Books.

Krishnan, V., Schoeffel, P. & Warren, J. (1994). Who goes where?. Wellington: New Zealand Institute for Social Research & Development. *The challenges of change: Pacific Island Communities in New Zealand 1986–1993* (pp. 9–25). Wellington, New Zealand: New Zealand Institute for Social Research & Development.

Madraiwiwi, J. (2008). *A personal perspective: The speeches of Joni Madraiwiwi*. Suva, Fiji: IPS Publications. University of the South Pacific.

Meo-Sewabu, L. & Walsh-Tapiata, W. (2012). Global declarations and village discourses: Social policy and indigenous wellbeing. *Alter Native Journal: Nga Pae o te Maramatanga, 8*(3), 305–317.

Nabobo-Baba, U. (2006). *Knowing and learning: An indigenous Fijian approach*. Suva, Fiji: Institute of Pacific Studies, USP.

Nabobo-Baba, U. (2008). Decolonising framings in Pacific Research: Indigenous Fijian Vanua Research Framework as an organic response. *Alter Native Journal: Nga Pae o te Maramatanga, 4*(2), 140–154.

Pabon, L., Umapathi, N. & Waqavonovono, E. (2012). How geographically concentrated is poverty in Fiji? *Asia Pacific Viewpoint, 53*(2), 205–217. doi: 10.1111/j.1467-8373.2012.01485.x

Putnam, R. D. (2000). *Bowling alone: The collapse and revival of American community*. New York, NY: Simon and Schuster.

Putnam, R. D., Leonardi, R. & Nanetti, R. (1993). *Making democracy work: Civic traditions in modern Italy*. Boston, MA: Princeton University Press.

Ratuva, S. (2010). Back to basics: Towards integrated social protection for vulnerable groups in Vanuatu. *Pacific Economic Bulletin, 25*(3), 40–63.

Rotuivaqali, M. T. (2012). *Evaluation of Fiji, Solomon Islands, and Vanuatu's social protection policies post 2008: Global Economic Crisis (GEC)*. Retrieved from www.gdn.int/admin/uploads/editor/files/2013Conf_Papers/MasilinaTuiloaRotuivaqali_paper.pdf

Spicker, P. (2014). *Social policy: Theory and practice* (3rd ed.). Bristol, United Kingdom: The Policy Press.

Spoonley, P. (2001). Transnational Pacific communities: Transforming the politics of place and identity. In C. McPherson, P. Spoonley & M. Anae (Eds.), *Tangata o te moana nui: The evolving identities of Pacific peoples in Aotearoa/New Zealand*. Palmerston North, New Zealand: Dunmore Press Ltd.

Statistics New Zealand. (2014). *New Zealand income survey-information releases*. Retrieved from www.stats.govt.nz/browse_for_stats/income-and-work/Income/nz-income-survey-info-releases.aspx

UN Women (2015). *Progress of the world's women 2015–2016: Transforming economies, realizing rights*. New York: UN Women.

United Nations Permanent Forum on Indigenous Issues (2009). *State of the world's Indigenous peoples*. New York: United Nations.

Veenstra, G. & Patterson, A. C. (2012). Capital relations and health: Mediating and moderating effects of cultural, economic, and social capitals on mortality in Almeda County, California. *International Journal of Health Services*, 42(2), 277–291.

Vertovec, S. (2009). *Transnationalism*. London: Routledge.

Vunidilo, K. (2008). *Living in two worlds: Challenges facing Pacific people in New Zealand: The case of Fijians living in Aotearoa, New Zealand*. Saarbrucken, Germany: VDM Verlag Dr. Muller Aktiengesellschaft & Company.

Suggested further readings/websites

Airhihenbuwa, C. O. (2010). Culture matters in global health. *The European Health Psychologist*, 12(December), 52–55.

Asian Development Bank. (2010). *Enhancing social protection in Asia and the Pacific: The proceedings of the regional workshop*. Retrieved from http://adb.org/sites/default/files/pub/2011/proceedings-enhancing-social-protection.pdf

Durie, M. (2004). Understanding health and illness: Research at the interface between science and indigenous knowledge. *International Journal of Epidemiology*, 33(5), 1138–1143. Retrieved from http://ije.oxfordjournals.org/content/33/5/1138.full.pdf

International Labour Organization. (2012). *Social Protection floor*. Retrieved from www.ilo.org/secsoc/areas-of-work/policy-development-and-applied-research/social-protection-floor/lang--en/index.htm

Meo-Sewabu, L. (2016). Na marama itaukei kei na vanua: Culturally embedded agency of indigenous Fijian women: Opportunities and constraints. *New Zealand Sociology*, 31(2), 96–122.

Mlambo-Ngcuka, P. (2015). Change is coming. Change has to come. *Commission on the Status of Women (CSW 59)*. Retrieved from www.unwomen.org/en/news/stories/2015/3/change-is-coming-change-has-to-come-executive-director

Ravuvu, A. (1983). *Vaka i taukei: The Fijian way of life*. Suva: Institute of Pacific Studies of the University of the South Pacific.

United Nations Permanent Forum on Indigenous Issues. (2009). *State of the World's Indigenous Peoples*. New York: United Nations.

PART III
Social policy

18
NAVIGATING SOCIAL POLICY PROCESSES IN THE PACIFIC

Leituala Kuiniselani Toelupe Tago-Elisara and Donald Bruce Yeates

Key points

- The social policy process in the Pacific is located within the wider public policy space and within a Pacific-Indigenous and regional institutional framework.
- Various organisations are working collaboratively to implement regional policy priorities at national and community levels.
- Social workers are encouraged to understand the process, navigate within and across policy sectors and engage the policy process at junctures which align with the context of their practice.

Introduction

Globally, the goals of social policy have broadened from meeting specific social sector goals (such as education) through the statutory provision of social services to addressing the complex sustainable development issues of poverty alleviation, social protection, social inclusion, the promotion of human rights and environmental justice (Hall, 2004). These broader goals were inherent in the Millennium Development Goals 2000–2015 and are now embedded in the Sustainable Development Goals (SDGs) 2016–2030 (Midgley & Pawar, 2017). Implementing these goals requires a multi-sectoral policy approach and the actions of the state, civil society, the private sector and international development institutions. The increasing "globalization" of social policy through development banks, United Nations bodies, regional and supranational organisations raises important issues in the Pacific about where "regional, national and local" social policy-making lies.

The purpose of policy research has been to create an understanding of the relationships and inter-actions between the institutions of government, political actors and the different population groups for whom these policies are intended (Petridou, 2014). This understanding is informed by several theories of the policy processes including an advocacy coalition framework, institutional analysis and development framework, and social construction and design (Aiafi, 2017). The contextual relevance of these theories to the Pacific is called into question as these contributions remain focused on North America and Europe (Adams, Minnichelli & Ruddell, 2014; Saetren, 2005).

The Pacific Islands Forum[1] is a political and economic policy making organisation that has over the years focused on and articulated broader public policy for the Pacific region (Pacific Islands Forum Secretariat, 2018d). This chapter seeks to explore the social policy process in the Pacific in the wider public policy space, and the importance of peak bodies and advocacy groups in supporting the mobilisation of change across the global, Pacific regional and national/local levels of society. Within a Pacific-Indigenous and regional institutional framework, it considers the role of various organisations that are working collaboratively to implement regional policy priorities at national and community levels. The development of the Pacific Platform for Action on Gender Equality and Women's Human Rights 2018–2030 provides social workers an instance of how the regional social policy process works. Social workers are encouraged to understand the process, navigate within and across policy sectors and engage the policy process at junctures which align with the context of their practice.

Social policy: a Pacific-Indigenous and regional institutional framework

The history and journey of Pacific people, in the context of "colonization, modernization and neo-colonial influences, have had a significant impact on the development of social policies and in turn a considerable impact on the cultural wellbeing of indigenous people" (Meo-Sewabu & Walsh-Tapiata, 2012, p. 305). It has been suggested that this history has resulted in the colonisation of minds of Pacific people and that for Pacific people to be able to take advantage of the "reservoirs of knowledge and practice that are our heritage, ... we [need to] collectively commit ourselves to re-constructing or re-fashioning our own epistemologies [otherwise] the risk is that others will define us" (Madraiwiwi, 2008, p. 4).

While these outside impacts still have an effect on policy making, Pacific people across the region are now at the helm of their own *va'a* (Samoan for canoe) or *vaka* (Fijian and Maori for canoe) navigating through development and making strides towards achieving their aspirations and goals. Meo-Sewabu and Walsh-Tapiata (2012) and Madraiwiwi (2008) describe a shift in consciousness amongst Pacific people that recognises the importance of their own voice and their knowledge in identifying solutions to the many social challenges and adversities that are faced. This shift also speaks to the notion that we ought to be looking "within" for solutions that ensures our wellbeing (Meo-Sewabu &

Walsh-Tapiata, 2012), and those that will protect and sustain our cultures and systems of knowledge.

Three key goals underpin an indigenous policy perspective: participation, indigeneity and equality (Durie, 2005). Broad policies emerging from these goals are: 1) Full participation in society, education and the economy (the participatory goal); 2) Certainty of access to indigenous culture, networks and resources by indigenous peoples (the indigeneity goal); and 3) Fairness between members of society (the equality goal). Indigenous policies also need to recognise collectives as fundamental to society.

The Framework for Pacific Regionalism (Pacific Islands Forum Secretariat, 2014) sets out a regional priority policy setting process that is consultative in nature. The process is meant to be inclusive of all stake holders and involves a flow of proposals from the local/national level through to the Forum Secretariat, vetted by a Forum Officials' Committee (FOC) and submitted to the Forum Leaders' meetings for final regional policy decision-making and over-sight. Existing Forum Ministerial and Officials' meetings are integrated in this process. With these regional policy priorities, national and local stakeholders are able to align national policies and resources to achieve the goals of the regional priorities.

The "Blue Pacific" identity adopted by the Leaders in 2017 emphasised collective action for communal wellbeing through a development process that is planned, owned and based on the needs and potential of the peoples of the Pacific (Pacific Islands Forum Secretariat, 2018c). The Blue Pacific symbolises the diverse cultures of the Pacific Islands and provides "An identity that is grounded in something as vast as the sea ... [that exercises] ... our minds and rekindle[s] in us the spirit that sent our ancestors to explore the oceanic unknown and make it their home, our home" (Hau'ofa, 2008, p. 42). The Blue Pacific focuses policy on the environment and the Ocean's resources and geography. Through the Framework, Pacific leaders both align regional policies to the global development agenda and through a united front inform and influence international development agendas (Pacific Islands Forum Secretariat, 2018b).

The social policy process in the Pacific is multifaceted and multi-layered (Pacific Islands Forum Secretariat, 2017). The various components of the process are outlined in Figure 18.1.

The first layer denotes the global policy agendas such as the 2030 Sustainable Development Agenda. The second layer identifies the Small Island Developing States (SIDS) global agenda. Thirteen Pacific countries[2] are members of the United Nations (UN) SIDS, a grouping of states deemed to have "their own peculiar [sustainable development] vulnerabilities and characteristics" (United Nations, Division for Sustainable Development Goals, DESA, 2018, para. 1). The third layer focuses on the Pacific and the Framework for Pacific Regionalism. Within the Pacific region there are the sector policy frameworks as indicated in the fourth layer. National development and sector policies and strategies follow at the fifth layer with the translation of policies into local programmes and projects at the sixth layer and project implementation in communities at the seventh layer.

1. Global Agendas
2. Global Agenda: Small Island Developing States
3. Framework For Pacific Regionalism
4. Pacific Regional Sector Policy Frameworks
5. National Development and Sector Policies and Strategies
6. Local Programmes and Projects
7. Community Project Implementation

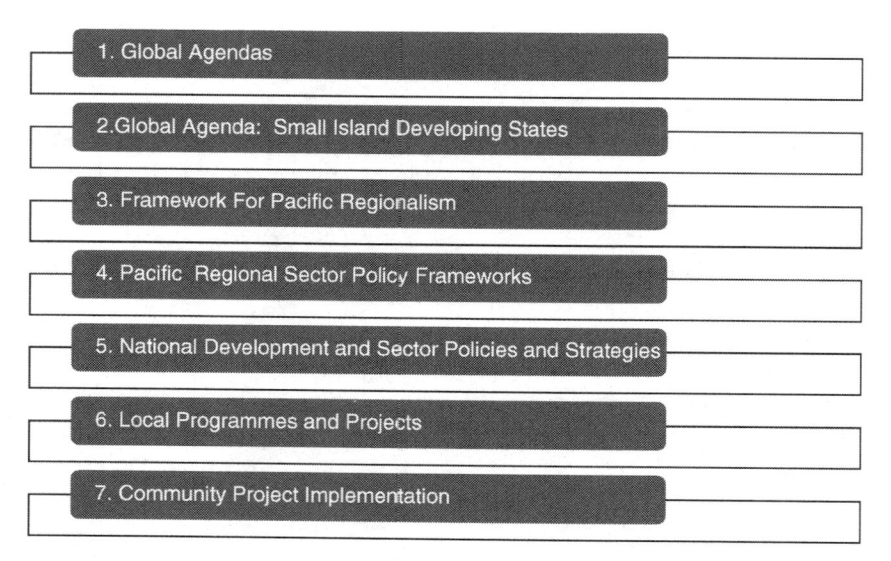

FIGURE 18.1   Social policy process in the Pacific.

The policy framework for the Pacific is symbolic of the ebbs and flows of these different layers and how each one serves to inform each other through both a bottom up and top down approach in practice.

Roles of government, regional and civil society/non-government organisations

At the national level, the 22 Pacific Island Countries and Territories (PICTs) of the Secretariat of the Pacific Community (SPC)[3] have developed their own frameworks, models and practices of developing social policies and public policies to suit their political, economic, social and cultural contexts. This means that PICTs are at different levels and stages in social policy development, analysis and practice. Their diverse contexts warrants that each should be considered uniquely from a geo-political and socio-economic perspective.

At the regional level, the Council of Regional Organisations of the Pacific (CROP)[4] functions as a coordination mechanism to provide policy advice and may assist in facilitating policy formulation at the national, regional and international level (Pacific Islands Forum Secretariat, 2018e). Policy advice and policy formulation support provided by the various CROP agencies are often a response to a call for:

1. coordination in regard to the regional development agenda;
2. translating global policy agendas to the Pacific context; and
3. Pacific positioning relative to policy discussions at the inter-regional or global level.

(Author's construct based on literature and current practice)

Based on these parameters of policy support for PICTs, the role of CROP agencies is critical in enabling the regional policy landscape across the different sectors of development. Individual CROP agencies regularly convene government meetings across the Pacific to consult on regional policy issues. These regional meetings have resulted in several policy frameworks that guide the work of the different sectors both at national, regional and international levels. This convening capacity of CROP has expanded the meetings from targeting those in Governments and the public sector to include the private sector and Civil Society Organisations (CSOs). The CSO Engagement Strategy defines the roles, outlines the processes and principles for joint engagement and recognises "the need for a more coherent and coordinated approach to engagement" in the regional policy process (Pacific Islands Forum Secretariat, 2016). Several regional policy frameworks[5] which fall within the third and fourth levels of the Framework in Figure 18.1 have been produced as a result of these regional dialogues. The policy frameworks guide decision making and provide the basis for resource mobilisation and programme development and implementation across PICTs.

At the global level, the engagement of civil society organisations (CSOs) and non-government organisations (NGOs) has become a positive trend in the development space (Tortajada, 2016). Who participates as legitimate parties in the Pacific policy process continues to evolve. The role of CSOs in policy analysis, formulation and implementation through the delivery of services for PICTs has become more noticeable. This prominence is due in part to the fact that Pacific governments are challenged with financial and human resource constraints. This change also recognises the expertise that CSOs/NGOs bring to the table, which address the social policy issues and the developmental challenges PICTs face (Pacific Islands Forum Secretariat, 2016).

Social policy implementation and practice

Social policy implementation in the Pacific is characterised by strategies from multiple sectors targeted to meet the needs of different population groups. Cross-sectoral integration of policy development has resulted in creating synergies across sectors, eliminating duplication and coordinating approaches for sustainable development. This shift in practice has not come without challenges. Policy makers often lack an understanding and appreciation of social policy analysis in achieving development outcomes. In addressing this issue, the SPC adopted a systematic approach to educating key stakeholders and provided direct technical support in integrating a social policy analysis and perspective across the SPC's scientific and technical programmes (Braun, 2012).

An important component of the support provided is the training in data collection used as evidence to inform the integration of social policy analysis across sectors. Mainstreaming gender analysis has facilitated an appreciation of the need for gender statistics in promoting gender equality (Pacific Community, 2018b). Gender analysis contributes to evidence-based policies and decision-making and the subsequent development of appropriate interventions that respond to the needs of men and women and different population groups at all levels. The conduct of family safety studies (see, for example, Ali, 2006; UN Women, 2015; Pacific Community, 2018a) has resulted in the development of legislation aimed at ending domestic violence and has generated some support for the creation of shelters and services for women and children victims. Developing the necessary services catering for the needs of the victims and perpetrators of violence continues to be a gap in policy implementation (Pacific Community, 2018a). Generating data and statistical analysis to inform social policies and monitor their effectiveness and impact continues to be an issue across the PICTs (Pacific Community, 2018b).

The provision of social services by Pacific government departments is the main means of social policy implementation and focus for social work practice. The role of government in providing the public services for health and education remains. CSOs/NGOs or Community Based Organisations (CBOs) are being tasked with the provision of social services either through targeted interventions or through integrated service delivery. CBOs are involved in rolling out community development services depending on the infrastructure and social structures that exist. Shelters and crisis centres for victims of violence are more likely to be provided by CSOs/NGOs such as the Samoa Victims Support, the Women and Children Crisis Centre in Tonga and the Fiji Women's Crisis Centre. Formal social protection and welfare support are limited to national provident funds and social security systems primarily for those in formal employment. Some countries also provide universal non-contributory pension schemes for the elderly, disability benefits and grants targeting children, including for some a one-off lump sum payment for newborns and infants (Pacific Community, 2018c).

Traditional forms of social protection continue to provide safety nets for PICTs, including social work often delivered as part of community development services by clan and extended family or village community structures. The kinship system, referred to as *veiwekani* in Fiji, *fa'a Samoa* in Samoa or *wantok* in PNG and the Solomon Islands, sustains individuals and families on a daily or occasional basis (International Labour Organization, 2006). Communities have utilised these kinship systems and social structures to address social challenges and create solutions from resources embedded in their social and cultural contexts. Growing urbanisation and migration have resulted in weakened family ties. The gradual erosion of traditional forms of social protection has left an increasing proportion of the population in PICTs more vulnerable to social and economic pressures (International Labour Organization, 2006).

Social workers need to leverage regional and global social policy in their practice to affect change at the community and national level in the context in which they work. Their practice experience affords them the opportunity to inform and influence policy development at the Pacific regional and global levels. The story of the development of the Pacific Platform for Action on Gender Equality and Women's Human Rights 2018–2030 (Pacific Community, 2017) can assist one in understanding the policy process and leverage policy in practice and influence policy development.

Pacific platform for action on gender equality and women's human rights 2018–2030 context

The SPC coordinated and convened a PICTs' preparatory meeting prior to their engagement and participation at the 1994 Fourth World Conference for Women held in Beijing, China (the Beijing Conference). Twelve areas of concern for gender equality and women's empowerment in the Pacific were generated from this meeting: health, education and training, economic empowerment, agriculture and fishing, legal and human rights, shared decision-making, environment, culture and the family, mechanisms to promote the advancement of women, violence, peace and justice, poverty and indigenous people's rights. These concerns were then adopted as the Pacific Platform for Action (PPA) on the Advancement of Women and Gender Equality, which essentially mirrored the critical areas of concern outlined in the Beijing Platform for Action. The rationale behind having a regional platform in addition to the global platform (the Beijing Platform for Action) was to include issues of particular relevance to the Pacific and to embed a Pacific context (Pacific Community, 2015). The PPA has undergone two major reviews that have resulted in a renewed approach to the PPA, taking into account the changing geo-political, social, economic and cultural context of PICTs and more importantly, the changing policy landscape and development space in the Pacific.

Target audience

The focus of the PPA is Pacific women and girls and applies to CROP, PICTs Governments and Administrations, CSOs/NGOs, Development Partners, private sector organisations and the faith-based sector.

Policy development process

Governments of PICTs and CSOs were engaged in the development and review of the policy. Through the convening powers of SPC, these stakeholders were provided an opportunity to contribute to the discussions during various stages of the process – from the start of the initial conversation in 1994 through to the implementation, monitoring, reviews and the reformulation of the Policy Framework 2018–2030. The key elements for consideration throughout all phases included:

- the need to embed Pacific context and Pacific - Indigenous perspectives;
- alignment to relevant global and national level policy frameworks. This is important in realising synergies across regional policies and as a coordinated approach to addressing gender equality issues in the region;
- an inclusive process that engaged all sectors in the consultations – public, private, CSO and church sectors and women of all diversities;
- the framework needed to be responsive to the changing context and to the needs of women and girls across the Pacific;

- that it was regularly monitored and reviewed towards adapting the framework and taking into consideration the learning from lessons over time;
- the policy also needed to provide a balance between taking an approach that targeted and focused delivery on specific populations and taking an approach that integrated and mainstreamed gender equality and women's human rights across policy sectors.

Progress

The PPA on Gender Equality and Women's Human Rights 2018–2030 was endorsed at the Thirteenth Conference of Pacific Women and the Sixth Meeting of the Pacific Ministers for Women (Pacific Community, 2016). The renewed PPA seeks to assist PICTs in accelerating the implementation of all its gender equality commitments and takes into account other recent developments in the global and regional policy space for gender equality in the Pacific. Regional coordination in general is a challenging task given the many players in the development arena, their competing agendas and PICTs competing priorities.

Conclusion

The social policy process in the Pacific is centred at the regional institutional level through the Framework for Pacific Regionalism. The process also evolves around the relevant regional sector policy frameworks focused on targeted interventions to address development challenges for Pacific people. The Regional Policy Framework allows Pacific governments to align and integrate national policies and resources to achieve the goals of the regional priorities. Pacific governments are able to align regional and national policies to global agendas while presenting a Pacific-Indigenous collective stance in international arenas informing and influencing global decision-making. CSOs have become increasingly engaged in the policy process although capacity issues pose barriers to their full participation. The mandated responsibilities of the various CROP agencies are critical in the process providing policy advice, support for policy formulation and scientific and technical support. Social workers in the Pacific need to understand this policy process, be conscious of the need to navigate within and across sectors, and be engaged in the community, national, regional and global levels of the process.

Notes

1 The PIF comprises 18 members: Australia, Cook Islands, Federated States of Micronesia, Fiji, French Polynesia, Kiribati, Nauru, New Caledonia, New Zealand, Niue, Palau, Papua New Guinea, Republic of Marshall Islands, Samoa, Solomon Islands, Tonga, Tuvalu and Vanuatu.
2 SIDS Pacific members: Fiji, Kiribati, Marshall Islands, Micronesia (Federated States of), Nauru, Palau, Papua New Guinea, Samoa, Solomon Islands, Timor-Leste, Tonga, Tuvalu, Vanuatu.

3 The SPC is an international scientific and technical development organisation serving the Pacific region. The PICTs members are: American Samoa, Cook Islands, Fiji, French Polynesia, Guam, Kiribati, Marshall Islands, Federated States of Micronesia, Nauru, New Caledonia, Niue, Northern Mariana Islands, Palau, Papua New Guinea, Pitcairn Islands, Samoa, Solomon Islands, Tokelau, Tonga, Tuvalu, Vanuatu, Wallis and Futuna (Pacific Community, 2018).
4 CROP agencies are: Forum Fisheries Agency; Pacific Aviation Safety Office; Pacific Power Association; Pacific Islands Development Programme; Pacific Community–SPC; Secretariat of the Pacific Regional Environmental Programme; South Pacific Tourism Organisation and The University of the South Pacific. The Pacific Islands Forum Secretariat acts as CROP's permanent chair and provides secretariat support.
5 Some specific examples of these regional policy frameworks are: the Pacific Leaders Gender Equality Declaration (Pacific Islands Forum Secretariat, 2012); the Pacific Platform for Action for Gender Equality and Women's Human Rights (Pacific Community, 2017); the Pacific Youth Development Framework (Pacific Community – SPC, 2017); and the Pacific Regional Education Development Framework (Pacific Island Forum Secretariat, 2018a).

References

Adams, W. C., Minnichelli, L. F. & Ruddell, M. W. (2014). Policy journal trends and tensions: JPAM and PSJ. *Policy Studies Journal, 42*, 118–137.

Aiafi, R. P. (2017). The nature of public policy processes in the Pacific Islands. *Asia and the Pacific Policy Studies, 4*(3), 451–466. https://doi.org/10.1002/app5.196

Ali, S. (2006). *Violence against the girl child in the Pacific Islands region*. Florence, Italy: United Nations Division for the Advancement of Women.

Braun, T. (Ed.) (2012). *Stocktake of gender mainstreaming capacity of Pacific Island governments – Federated States of Micronesia*. Noumea, New Caledonia: Secretariat of the Pacific Community.

Durie, M. (2005). Race and ethnicity in public policy: Does it work. *Social Policy Journal of New Zealand, 24*, 1–11.

Hall, M. (2004). *Social policy for development*. London: Sage Publications.

Hau'ofa, E. (2008). *We are the ocean*. Honolulu, HI: University of Hawai'i Press.

International Labour Organization. (2006). *Social protection for all men and women: A source book for extending social security in Fiji*. Suva, Fiji: International Labour Organization.

Madraiwiwi, J. (2008). *A personal perspective: The speeches of Joni Madraiwiwi*. Suva, Fiji: ISP Publications, The University of the South Pacific.

Meo-Sewabu, L. & Walsh-Tapiata, W. (2012). Global declarations and village discourse: Social policy and indigenous wellbeing. *AlterNative: An International Journal of Indigenous Peoples, 8*(3), 304–317.

Midgley, J. & Pawar, M. (Eds.). (2017). *Future directions in social development*. New York: Palgrave Macmillan.

Pacific Community. (2015). *Review of Pacific platform for action on empowerment of women and gender equality*. Noumea, New Caledonia: Pacific Community.

Pacific Community. (2016). *Outcomes of the 13th Triennial Conference of Pacific Women and the 6th Meeting of the Pacific Ministers for Women*. Suva, Fiji: Pacific Community.

Pacific Community. (2017). *Pacific Platform for Action on Gender Equality and Women's Human Rights 2018–2030*. Retrieved from www.spc.int/updates/blog/2017/10/new-road-map-fast-track-gender-equality

Pacific Community. (2018). *Brief on poverty alleviation and social protection*. Noumea, New Caledonia: Pacific Community.

Pacific Community. (2018a). *Changing laws, protecting women project*. Retrieved from http://rrrt.spc.int/projects/violence-against-women
Pacific Community. (2018b). *Gender and culture statistics*. Retrieved from http://sdd.spc.int/en/stats-by-topic/gender-and-culture-statistics
Pacific Community. (2018c). *Our members*. Retrieved from www.spc.int/our-members/
Pacific Community – SPC. (2017). *Pacific youth development framework*. Suva, Fiji: Secretariat of the Pacific Community.
Pacific Islands Forum Secretariat. (2012). *Pacific leaders gender equality declaration*. Suva, Fiji: Pacific Islands Forum Secretariat.
Pacific Islands Forum Secretariat. (2014). *Framework for Pacific regionalism*. Suva, Fiji: Pacific Islands Forum Secretariat.
Pacific Islands Forum Secretariat. (2016). *Civil society organisations engagement strategy*. Suva, Fiji: Pacific Islands Forum Secretarait.
Pacific Islands Forum Secretariat. (2017). *Pacific roadmap for sustainable development*. Suva, Fiji: Pacific Islands Forum Secretariat.
Pacific Island Forum Secretariat. (2018a). *Draft Pacific regional education development framework 2018 –2030*. Suva, Fiji: Pacific Islands Forum Secretariat.
Pacific Islands Forum Secretariat. (2018b). *Pacific leadership on ocean management and conservation*. Retrieved from www.forumsec.org/pacific-leadership-on-ocean-management-and-conservation/
Pacific Islands Forum Secretariat. (2018c). *Pacific regionalism and the blue Pacific*. Retrieved from Pacific Islands Forum Secretariat: www.forumsec.org/pacific-regionalism/
Pacific Islands Forum Secretariat. (2018d). *Who we are – Pacific Islands forum*. Retrieved from www.forumsec.org/who-we-arepacific-islands-forum/
Pacific Islands Forum Secretariat. (2018e). *Who we work with: Council of regional organisations of the Pacific*. Retrieved from www.forumsec.org/council-of-regional-organisations-of-the-pacific/
Petridou, E. (2014). Theories of the policy process: Contemporary scholarship and future directions. *Policy Studies Journal, 42*, s12–s32.
Saetren, H. (2005). Facts and myths about research on public policy implementation: Out-of-fashion, allegedly dead, but still very much alive and relevant. *Policy Studies Journal, 33*(4), 559–582.
Tortajada, C. (2016). Non-government organisations in global public policy. *Asia and Pacific Policy Studies Journal, 3*(2), 266–274.
UN Women. (2015). *How to design projects to end violence against women and girls. A step-by-step guide to taking action*. Suva, Fiji: UN Women Pacific Multi-Country Office.
United Nations, Division for Sustainable Development Goals DESA. (2018, October 23). *Small island developing states*. Retrieved from https://sustainabledevelopment.un.org/topics/sids

PART IV
Research

19
TOWARDS A PACIFIC-INDIGENOUS RESEARCH PARADIGM FOR PACIFIC SOCIAL WORK

Tracie Mafile'o, Peter Mataira and Kate Saxton

Key points

- Pacific social work research and evaluation approaches ought to align with a Pacific-Indigenous research paradigm.
- A Pacific-Indigenous research paradigm includes assumptions about reality, knowledge, values and methodologies from within Pacific worldviews.
- Pacific research approaches are increasingly being applied in research with Pacific communities, including: *kakala, vanua, talanoa* and *fa'afaletui*.
- The Strengths Enhancing Evaluation Research (SEER) approach is an example of the application of Pacific-Indigenous evaluation in Hawai'i.
- Decolonisation and positionality are important processes and considerations in Pacific research.

Introduction

Research informs social work practice, programmes and policy to achieve social justice and wellbeing. The research and evaluation approaches employed in Pacific social work, however, can work to silence or bring forth Pacific knowledges and ways. Research paradigms comprise assumptions about reality, knowledge, the role of values and methodologies. This chapter advocates a Pacific-Indigenous research paradigm to benefit Pacific health and social service users and communities. The first section discusses the context of Pacific research and considers decolonisation, diversity and the need for Pacific-led developmental research. Select Pacific-Indigenous research methodologies are then overviewed (*Kakala, Vanua, Talanoa* and *Fa'afaletui*) as a basis for proposing a Pacific-Indigenous research paradigm. To illustrate the application of Pacific-Indigenous social work research, the last section shares two specific research stories. The first is the Strengths Enhancing Evaluation Research (SEER) as an evaluation approach with āina-based (land-based) programmes in Hawaii. The second is a story about social work practice research in Fiji and how decolonisation and positionality was navigated.

Context of Pacific social work research

"Research" and "social work" are politically and culturally laden terms. Research is associated with the Western scientific tradition, while social work has roots within Western enlightenment responses to the industrial revolution in Europe and Northern America. Both research and social work are complicit in coloniality across Oceania and indeed globally (Fejo-King & Mataira, 2015; Johnson & Yellow Bird, 2012). Many scholars, including Pacific writers, have critiqued western research which justified colonisation and the subjugation of indigenous knowledges and people (Chilisa, 2012; Nabobo-Baba, 2008; Smith, 2012). Pacific social work research claims Pacific-Indigenous space in both research and social work traditions, whilst acknowledging that legitimacy stems from Pacific-Indigenous knowledge systems and cosmologies outside of "Enlightenment" and the industrial revolution. Contemporary Pacific social work research navigates the tensions between old and new in a context of ongoing coloniality (Carranza, 2018; Mignolo, 2011), and seeks to innovate and create new Indigenous knowledge (Royal, 2002). An example of such new knowledge is the Pacific Identity and Wellbeing Scale, a tool for incorporating measures of wellbeing based on Pacific cultural conceptions and Pacific realities (Manuela & Anae, 2017). Pacific social work research acknowledges the persistence of Pacific cultural knowledge and values over time, whilst accounting for the changing way in which Pacific culture is expressed.

Pacific hyper-diversity has implications for research. Research undertaken with communities in the diaspora, such as Tongan families in Los Angeles for example, may not translate well, if at all, to practice issues and concerns with Tongan families in Tonga. Research must also consider diverse perspectives when researching amongst cultures with hierarchical structures where speaking rights are traditionally assigned accordingly. Furthermore, whilst this discussion focuses on Pacific-Indigenous research, there is a need to support non-Western epistemologies of diverse Pacific populations more generally, including those linked to experiences of indentured labour in the Fiji context. The current reality is that most research is undertaken, or at least reported, using the English language. Arguably, Pacific research conducted fully in English can entail a form of neo-colonialism and raises challenges for researchers around translation processes and use of power in research processes. Ethnic specific disaggregation of data is another important consideration. For example, data collection with "Pacific" as an ethnic category will not show the differences between specific ethnic groups (for example, Cook Islands, Fiji or Nauru) in their experiences of elder care, youth offending or language retention, for example. If social programming is to be viable and well targeted to address community need, knowledge is needed about the differences amongst Pacific groups. Ethnic-specific language and cultural diversity is an important consideration for Pacific social work research to be both collaborative and empowering.

Pacific-led research is an important consideration given global disparity in knowledge-production between North and South, and between well-resourced and less-resourced contexts (Mafile'o, 2016). As the Pacific and its people have been largely studied by non-Pacific scholars, research and services "by Pacific for Pacific" is widely advocated (Health Research Council of New Zealand, 2014; Robie, 2018). Mutual research capacity strengthening (Redman-MacLaren et al., 2012) is a precursor for transformative Pacific-led research in social work. How data is used and translated, and by whom, into effective policy and then to action requires strong messaging, strategic alignment and political influence.

Developmental Pacific social work research, which benefits Pacific families and communities, is a priority; it is not enough to gain knowledge for the sake of knowing. While social work strongly advocates for social justice, in effect, its interventions have been inadequate to address economic injustice for marginalised Pacific communities. To achieve sustainable development, Pacific social work research must then be cognisant of the consequences of economic (under)development on Pacific families and communities. Unless research speaks directly to policy-makers about Pacific-Indigenous economic investment and resourcing to improve wellbeing, no amount of evidence or collaboration will make a long-term difference.

Pacific-Indigenous research approaches

Pacific-Indigenous research approaches are increasingly employed in contemporary scholarship (for example: Anae, & Mila-Schaaf, 2010; Fa'avae, Jones, & Manu'atu, 2016; Health Research Council of New Zealand, 2014; Meo-Sewabu, 2014a, 2014b; Nabobo-Baba, 2008; Sanga & Reynolds, 2017; Smith, 2012; Suaalii-Sauni & Fulu-Aiolupotea, 2014; Vaioleti, 2006). Pacific-Indigenous research approaches add to a global movement of Indigenous scholarships advocating for the decolonisation of research and the articulation of Indigenous research paradigms (for example: Chilisa, 2012; Hart, 2010; Pidgeon, 2018).

The *Kakala* framework (Johansson Fua, 2014), originally developed by Tongan Professor Konai Helu Thaman (Thaman, 1997), uses the garland-making process as a metaphor for research. The first stage is *teu*, the preparation stage, in which research conceptualisation (why, who, what) takes place. Second, *toli*, the careful and negotiated selection of flowers for the garland, represents data collection. Next is *tui*, or stringing the garland, akin to identifying patterns in the data through analysis and negotiation of more data where needed. *Luva*, meaning giving a gift with "heartfelt sincerity, humility and honour" (Johansson Fua, 2014), refers to the research process in which the gift of knowledge is returned to those who had given the knowledge (Johansson Fua, 2014, p. 54). *Malie*, which in Tongan refers to an appreciative response from an audience, refers to the constant monitoring of research process for its utility, application and relevancy. Finally, *mafana*, referring to something which is heartfelt, is the final evaluation of research impact. The *Kakala* framework is guided by particular Pacific concepts and realities which give light to a process for knowledge generation.

Fiji *I'Taukei* (Indigenous) scholars have developed *Vanua*, a word referring to "the land", as a research approach (Meo-Sewabu, 2014a; Meo-Sewabu, 2015; Nabobo-Baba, 2008; Vudiniabola, 2011). Nabobo-Baba (2008) explains that the *Vanua* research framework is embedded in an Indigenous Fijian world view of the "interconnectedness of people to their land, environment, cultures, relationships, spirit world, beliefs, knowledge systems, values and God(s)" (p. 143). *Vanua* research principles are: (1) research benefits the researched; (2) knowledge is influenced by cultural values, protocols; (3) research indigenous language fluency; (4) Indigenous principle researchers; (5) respect and reciprocity, acknowledging Vanua structures and protocols; (6) building local research capacity; (7) accountability and meaningful feedback to community; and (8) Vanua and village chiefs and elders' permission for research (Nabobo-Baba, 2008). As an example of *Vanua* research in practice, Meo-Sewabu (2014a) developed a cultural discernment group to guide the research she undertook in her maternal village on Fiji women's views of wellbeing. She explains how the group advised on the cultural protocols required for engaging participants. This included gifting a *tabua* (whale tooth, highly valued and used in exchange and ceremony) and *yaqona* (plant root and drink). When "accepted by the village elders, it implies a blanket consent ... for all villagers to participate and support our work ... With this approval, individual consent was redundant" (Meo-Sewabu, 2014a, p. 351). Individual written consent, however, was expected by the academic institution. This example gives insight into how the *Vanua* research approach guides appropriate research protocol from an *I'Taukei* worldview, but also how this was negotiated to comply with requirements of academic institutions operating predominantly from a non-Indigenous perspective.

Talanoa (Fa'avae et al., 2016; Farrelly & Nabobo-Baba, 2014; Tunufa'i, 2016; Vaioleti, 2006; Vaka, Brannelly & Huntington, 2016) is a data collection method based on Pacific story-telling and the associated modes of engagement. Pacific and other researchers have used *Talanoa* as an alternative to either the individual or focus group interviewing. Unlike a focus group, where everyone is expected to verbally contribute, Vaka et al. (2016) note that in *Talanoa*, some participants may just offer nonverbal cues which encourage "speakers to keep on talking until they arrive at harmony (*mālie*) and warmth (*māfana*)" which sits within the *loto* [heart] to reveal "the essence and true opinions about the subject" (Vaka et al., 2016, p. 539). Caution has been raised about *Talanoa* being applied as a pan-Pacific method given that the concept carries meaning in just a few Pacific languages and cultures, which could be deemed as "colonising" in itself (Tunufa'i, 2016).

The *Fa'afaletui* approach, developed as a culturally appropriate research method to investigate Samoan perspectives on mental health issues (Tamasese et al., 2005), has since been more broadly adopted (McCarthy, Shaban & Stone, 2011; Suaalii-Sauni & Fulu-Aiolupotea, 2014). The *Fa'afaletui* is a method which captures a diversity of perspectives. Taking the metaphor of "many houses", community members in research exploring Samoan perspectives of mental health in New Zealand were divided into four houses or groups (elder women, elder men, young women and young men). Each group had separate discussions, then the perspectives of each group were brought together to negotiate a shared understanding on the topic. The *Fa'afaletui* approach incorporated the different experiences and views of mental health from island-born elders, but also allowed women's perspectives and those of youth to be freely offered.

While this discussion of Pacific research approaches is by no means exhaustive, Table 19.1 summarises assumptions underpinning the Pacific research approaches, suggesting components of a Pacific-Indigenous research paradigm.

In summary, there has been a proliferation of academic and scholarly work expanding, debating and supporting Pacific-Indigenous research approaches which together suggest the existence of a Pacific-Indigenous research paradigm

TABLE 19.1 Pacific-Indigenous research paradigm: Ontology, epistemology, axiology and methodology

Ontological assumptions	*Epistemological assumptions*	*Axiological assumptions*	*Methodological assumptions*
What is the nature of reality? What is real?	*What counts as knowledge? How are knowledge claims justified?*	*What is the role of values?*	*What is the process of research? What is the language of research?*
• Interconnectedness of human, environment and spiritual • Reality exists in the context of relationships with the temporal and transcendent worlds	• Oral, visual, and environmental repositories and transmission of knowledge privileged • Some knowledge is sensitive and sacred and not for all • Knowledge to benefit Pacific families and the wider communities	• Collective values lived out in everyday life and expressed in ceremony explicitly inform and guide research	• Pacific leadership and community ownership of research process • Engages cultural structures, processes and protocols for knowledge generation and dissemination • Pacific-Indigenous languages advocated as the primary language research takes place in

with assumptions related to reality, knowledge, values and research. Two research stories are presented next to illustrate applied Pacific social work research.

Research stories

Strengths Enhancing Evaluation Research (SEER) for land-based programmes (Hawaii)

Strengths Enhancing Evaluation Research (SEER) was developed at the University of Hawai'i, Myron B. Thompson School of Social Work, by Dr. Peter Mataira and Dr. Paula Morelli in response to changing perceptions, attitudes and feelings among Native Hawaiians about the nature and frustrations of doing standardised measurements in programme evaluations (SEER video can be viewed at: https://youtu.be/GEubejt8oUg). It is not a prescriptive method to doing evaluation research with Indigenous (Native Hawaiian) land-based programmes, but a way to resist determining outcomes using tools that interrogate, intrude and serve no benefit to the community (Morelli & Mataira, 2010). It claims no magic formula to radically shift the dominant research paradigm. Rather, it promotes a way of conscientising and re-enabling communities to take back power and control (Mataira, Matsuoka & Morelli, 2005). SEER contrasts a more prescriptive evaluation research that often limits scope, direction and intentionality. It invites a combination of methodologies beyond mixed or multi-research designs to more relational systems frameworks. As such, SEER:

- Opens pathways to communities to determine what research means to them and how it looks on the ground.
- Gives communities the time, space, scope and opportunity to discuss their own understanding of evidence and outcomes.
- Respects and honours the collective community spirit and people's relational connections to each other, to land, and their cultures.
- Recognises the responsibilities of researchers as "invited" guests and to respect community boundaries.
- Affirms knowledge sources on how, what, why, and when are embedded throughout the community.
- Opens lines of communications before, during and after studies are conducted.
- Establishes a clear understanding on who owns data, who has access to it and how it is to be used.
- Ensures publications resulting from research are jointly co-authored with key community people.
- Advocates for a human subjects approval process to be set up by and for communities.

Decolonised Pacific research methodologies and the principles and guidelines offered by SEER can be a start point to ensuring data remains sacred and people's rights are protected. Honouring traditions and acknowledging ones "guesthood" (Harvey, 2003) is critical and a vital means to respecting boundaries. Culturally responsive, Pacific-led research works in the best interests of everyone when there is mutual buy-in, an alignment of goals, an openness to addressing and resolving internal and external conflicts, autonomy and when communities see and feel a part of the process. When they are engaged and empowered they are the key decolonising agents in research.

For Pacific peoples, research as an endeavour is both venerated and vilified. It is set against a backdrop of a painful colonial past, and against prevalent social realities that include poverty and economic marginalisation. SEER is a product and a process and its premise is tied to the systematic dismantling of power structures and giving emphasis to community's right to reclaim their authority to decide. It acknowledges their resistance to "buying" into a system that has perpetually marginalised and invalidated who they are and what they know. There has to be recognition that collective Pacific cultures have inherent social and ecological orientations (McGregor et al., 2003) which have led to the development of highly sophisticated social economies and mechanisms for sustainable living and balanced prosperity. In research, there are two types of failure. As Karlan and Appel (2016) note, there is a failure "to research" – that is, when studies are conceived with a particular set of questions but do not manage to answer them in part or in whole. This can be because researchers begin with a faulty premise or a misguided design plan. While these may be technical or theoretical in nature, it is inherently a failure of a Western methodological bias. A second reason is not based on a flawed research design but because of a fundamental flaw in ideas; simply put, western traditions of research are inherently assumptive and predicated on values, beliefs and attitudes regarding whose methods matter, who controls the process and who must yield to power. SEER's intention is to mitigate these by being open, transparent and aware of ethical and moral considerations to decolonising research. This can only work when mutual trust is built into the front end of the research relationship.

REFLECTIVE QUESTIONS

1. As a researcher, how does acknowledging your role as a "guest" obligate you to be ethically and morally responsible?
2. What did you learn from watching the SEER video? What was helpful for doing research in Pacific communities?

Decolonisation and positionality in social work practice research (Fiji)

This story reflects on complexities I (Kate Saxton) experienced undertaking a PhD in Fiji. I was enrolled in an Australian based university. I encountered issues of positionality, as a white female living as an expatriate in Fiji and working at The University of the South Pacific.

The PhD research topic began in response to my experience living and working as a social worker in both Fiji and Tonga. I observed a tension between more "traditional" models of social care and the impetus to embrace Western models of "best practice". This was particularly overt within Colonial institutions of social care such as hospitals and prison services, although seemingly less of a priority in community based settings. Initially, I hoped to contribute to a Fijian definition of social work and Code of Ethics in recognition of the ambiguity and debate in community regarding the use of the term. I felt that having a shared understanding of social work would be unifying for the community and provide clarity around the goals and purpose of social work in Fiji. I perceived this as an act of reciprocity by providing a tangible piece of work to share with local constituents. Whilst the reasoning behind this was well intentioned, what I failed to realise were the dangers of promoting the view of Fijians as a singular homogenous group. Such an approach fails to account for diversity amongst Pacific communities and reinforces the issues of cultural ignorance in pre-determining research agendas in Pacific contexts. This issue is also symptomatic of top-down Western academic approaches where students are required to provide the university with clear pre-determined research objectives rather than enabling more collaborative and deductive approaches to research design.

Fortunately, I was engaged in deliberate critical reflection as part of a commitment to culturally responsive practice and this enabled me to adapt the research project to better reflect the lived experiences of Fijian constituents. Another strength of the research design was the inclusion of a Pacific Academic on the supervisory team. Initially the research design had a heavy focus on individual interviews as this reflected the dominance of both my epistemological framework and positionality of the white male supervisory team. This approach failed to adequately account for power dynamics in the researcher/participant relationship or provide opportunities for culturally informed research methodologies to take centre stage. Again this highlights the privileging of Western academic thought in the construction of research agendas and contributes to a cross-cultural research environment where the researcher was researching 'on' rather than 'with' Fijian social workers (Farrelly & Nabobo-Baba, 2014). Conversely, the involvement of a Pacific academic enabled the researcher to consider a more Pacific appropriate method, namely *Talanoa*, to inform the research design and emphasises the importance of engaging with cultural mentors in contexts of outsider-insider research. By drawing on *Talanoa* as a method within Fiji-based research, I sought to value traditional models of knowing and actively limit the privileging of Western epistemology as the basis for which knowledge must be interpreted.

Farrelly and Nabobo-Baba (2014) suggest that *Talanoa* research is best carried out once periods of prolonged community engagement have occurred and where trust, mutual understanding and respect can be established. In this context, researchers living within the community or who have perceived legitimate community ties may have the advantage of "insider" positioning. In my experience, the time taken to establish meaningful relationships was at odds with pressures to meet deadlines and research milestones stipulated by the Australian University and funding sources. There was often a clash between the objective-orientated focus of the university and the relational-oriented imperative within the Fijian community. If social work research is to be genuine in its commitments to culturally responsive practices, consideration needs to be given to time required to establish meaningful relationships with local counterparts. Whilst universities and Western research institutions will ultimately have research outputs to strive towards, such a position encourages time-bound data collection imposed in an effort to meet Western notions of productivity. Again, acknowledgement needs to be given to the stark difference in epistemological reasoning between Western and Pacific Island methodologies (Ravulo, 2016). It is imperative that Pacific focused research avoids processes that are inherently biased towards Western practices, thus the parameters for fieldwork should be met with flexibility by university ethics committees (Meo-Sewabu, 2014b).

REFLECTIVE QUESTIONS

1. What potential challenges can you identify for social workers interested in pursuing research with Pacific communities?
2. What strategies did the researcher engage with to ensure more culturally responsive practice?
3. What could have been done better?

Conclusion

Pacific communities face unnerving challenges in addressing and critiquing the hegemonic dominance encoded into the traditions of Western research. Communities and researchers must reconceptualise what decolonisation means in the wake of proliferating social technologies, realignments in geo-political and social order, rises in sea levels, increasing wealth disparities, global pandemics, neoliberalism, fascism and metadata. Narratives that affirm binaries – whether they be social, political or ideological in nature – are giving way to more inclusive (w)holistic discursive discourses and acceptance of multiple truths, perspectives and realities. Pacific communities are manifestations of their genealogical lineages spanning vast oceans, and as collective economic powerhouses resulting from political presence on the world stage and nascent forms of indigenous innovation and entrepreneurship (de Bruin & Mataira, 2003). Collectively, Pacific cultures reflect a rich temporal and transcendent nature of the human condition. Approaches to Pacific research and evaluation which embrace ancestral traditions, protocols of welcome, sacred and spiritual ceremony and see value in reconciling tensions lead to a more robust, engaged and equitable research endeavour. Such approaches reflect a Pacific-Indigenous research paradigm comprised of Pacific views of reality, knowledge, values and research process. The goal is not to reject tools associated with Western traditions but to include and elevate Indigenous methodologies that can best authenticate Pacific experiences, validate Pacific practices and legitimise and extend Pacific knowledge.

References

Anae, M. & Mila-Schaaf, K. (2010). *Teu le va – Relationships across research and policy in Pasifika education: A collective approach to knowledge generation and policy development for action towards Pasifika education success.* Wellington, New Zealand: Ministry of Education.

Carranza, M. E. (2018). International social work: Silent testimonies of the coloniality of power. *International Social Work, 61*(3), 341–352. doi:10.1177/0020872816631598

Chilisa, B. (2012). *Indigenous research methodologies.* Thousand Oaks, CA: Sage.

de Bruin, A., & Mataira, P. (2003). Indigenous entrepreneurship. In A. D. Bruin & A. Dupuis (Eds.), *Entrepreneurship: New perspectives in a global age* (pp. 169–184). Aldershot, United Kingdom: Ashgate.

Fa'avae, D., Jones, A. & Manu'atu, L. (2016). Talanoa'i 'a e talanoa – Talking about talanoa: Some dilemmas of a novice researcher. *AlterNative: An International Journal of Indigenous Peoples, 12*(2), 138–150.

Farrelly, T. & Nabobo-Baba, U. (2014). Talanoa as empathic apprenticeship. *Asia Pacific Viewpoint, 55*(3), 319–330.

Fejo-King, C. & Mataira, P. J. (2015). *Expanding the conversation: International Indigenous social workers' insights into the use of Indigenist knowledge and theory in practice.* Torrens, Australia: Magpie Goose Publishing.

Hart, M. A. (2010). Indigenous worldviews, knowledge, and research: The development of an Indigenous research paradigm. *Journal of Indigenous Voices in Social Work, 1*(1), 1–16.

Harvey, G. (2003). Guesthood as ethical decolonising research method. *Numen, 50*(2), 125–146.

Health Research Council of New Zealand. (2014). *Pacific health research guidelines.* Auckland, New Zealand: Health Research Council of New Zealand.

Johansson Fua, S. (2014). Kakala research framework: A garland in celebration of a decade of rethinking education. In M. Otunuku, U. Nabobo-Baba, and S. Johansson-Fua (Eds.), *Of waves, winds and wonderful things: A decade of rethinking Pacific education* (pp. 50–60). Suva, Fiji: USP Press.

Johnson, J. T. & Yellow Bird, M. (2012). Indigenous peoples and cultural survival. In L. M. Healy & R. J. Link (Eds.), *Handbook of international social work: Human rights, development, and the global profession* (pp. 208–213). New York: Oxford University Press.

Karlan, D. S. & Appel, J. (2016). *Failing in the field: What we can learn when field research goes wrong.* Princeton, NJ: Princeton University Press.

Mafile'o, T. A. (2016). Strengthening research capacity in Oceania. *Social Dialogue, 15*, 18–20.

Manuela, S. & Anae, M. (2017). Pacific youth, acculturation and identity: The relationship between ethnic identity and well-being – New directions for research. *Pacific Dynamics: Journal of Interdisciplinary Research*, *1*(1), 129–147.

Mataira, P., Matsuoka, J. K. & Morelli, P. T. (2005). Issues and processes in Indigenous research. *Hūlili*, *2*(1), 35–46.

McCarthy, A., Shaban, R. & Stone, C. (2011). Fa'afaletui: A framework for the promotion of renal health in an Australian Samoan community. *Journal of Transcultural Nursing*, *22*(1), 55–62. doi:10.1177/1043659610387154

McGregor, D. P. P. T., Matsuoka, J. K., Rodenhurst, R., Kong, N. & Spencer, M. S. (2003). An ecological model of Native Hawaiian well-being. *Pacific Health Dialog*, *10*(2), 106–128.

Meo-Sewabu, L. (2014a). Cultural discernment as an ethics framework: An Indigenous Fijian approach. *Asia Pacific Viewpoint*, *55*(3), 345–354. doi:https://doi.org/10.1111/apv.12059

Meo-Sewabu, L. (2014b). Research ethics: An indigenous Fijian perspective. In C. Cocker & T. Hafford-Letchfield (Eds.), *Rethinking anti-discriminatory and anti-oppressive theories for social work practice* (pp. 108–122). Houndmills, United Kingdom: Palgrave Macmillan.

Meo-Sewabu, L. D. (2015). *'Tu ga na inima ka luvu na waqa': (The bail to get water out of the boat is in the boat yet the boat sinks): The cultural constructs of health and wellbeing amongst Marama iTaukei in a Fijian village in Lau and in a transnational Fijian community in Whanganui, Aotearoa*. (Social Policy PhD), Massey University, Palmerston North, New Zealand.

Mignolo, W. D. (2011). Geopolitics of sensing and knowing: On (de)coloniality, border thinking and epistemic disobedience. *Postcolonial Studies*, *14*(3), 273–283. doi:http://dx.doi.org/10.1080/13688790.2011.613105

Morelli, P. T. & Mataira, P. J. (2010). Indigenizing evaluation research: A long-awaited paradigm shift. *Journal of Indigenous Voices in Social Work*, *1*(2), 1–12.

Nabobo-Baba, U. (2008). Decolonising framings in Pacific Research: Indigenous Fijian vanua research framework as an organic response. *AlterNative: An International Journal of Indigenous Peoples*, *4*(2), 140–154. doi:10.1177/117718010800400210

Pidgeon, M. (2018). Moving between theory and practice within an Indigenous research paradigm. *Qualitative Research*. doi:org/10.1177/1468794118781380

Ravulo, J. (2016). Pacific epistemologies in professional social work practice, policy and research. *Asia Pacific Journal of Social Work & Development (Routledge)*, *26*(4), 191.

Redman-MacLaren, M., MacLaren David, J., Harrington, H., Asugeni, R., Timothy-Harrington, R., Kekeubata, E. & Speare, R. (2012). Mutual research capacity strengthening: A qualitative study of two-way partnerships in public health research. *International Journal for Equity in Health*, *11*(1), 79. doi:10.1186/1475-9276-11-79

Robie, D. (2018, 25 February). More frontline research 'by Pacific for Pacific' plea at climate summit. *Asia Pacific Report*.

Royal, T. A. C. (2002). *Indigenous worldviews: A comparative study: A report on research in progress*. Wellington, New Zealand: Winston Churchill Memorial Trust.

Sanga, K. & Reynolds, M. (2017). To know more of what it is and what it is not: Pacific research on the move. *Pacific Dynamics: Journal of Interdisciplinary Research*, *1*(2), 198–204.

Smith, L. T. (2012). *Decolonizing methodologies: Research and indigenous peoples* (2nd ed.). Dunedin, New Zealand: Otago University Press.

Suaalii-Sauni, T. & Fulu-Aiolupotea, S. M. (2014). Decolonising Pacific research, building Pacific research communities and developing Pacific research tools: The case of the talanoa and the faafaletui in Samoa. *Asia Pacific Viewpoint, 55*(3), 331–344. doi:10.1111/apv.12061

Tamasese, K., Peteru, C., Waldegrave, C. & Bush, A. (2005). Ole taeao afua, the new morning: A qualitative investigation into Samoan perspectives on mental health and culturally appropriate services. *Australian & New Zealand Journal of Psychiatry, 39*(4), 300–309.

Thaman, K. H. (1997). *Kakala: A concept of teaching and learning.* Paper presented at the Australian college of education National Conference, Cairns, Australia.

Tunufa'i, L. (2016). Pacific research: Rethinking the talanoa "methodology". *New Zealand Sociology, 31*(7), 227–239.

Vaioleti, T. M. (2006). Talanoa research methodology: A developing position of Pacific research. *Waikato Journal of Education, 12*, 21–34.

Vaka, S., Brannelly, T. & Huntington, A. (2016). Getting to the heart of the story: Using talanoa to explore Pacific mental health. *Issues in Mental Health Nursing, 37*(8), 537–544. doi:doi:10.1080/01612840.2016.1186253

Vudiniabola, A. T. (2011). *The Fijian diploma of nursing curriculum: An indigenous case study of a curriculum change.* (Nursing PhD), Massey University, Palmerston North, New Zealand.

PART V
Future directions

20

WHERE TO FROM HERE?

Integration of indigenous knowledges and practice in contemporary settings

Jioji Ravulo and Wheturangi Walsh-Tapiata

Key points

- The inclusion of indigenous perspectives as part of the global definition in social work should be meaningfully utilised across social work education, practice, policy and research.
- Indigenous world views have been devalued at the cost of privileging dominant western discourses; however, this should be challenged and revalued.
- The need to promote the decoloniality of social work as everyone's responsibility is part of creating a sustainable change and difference.
- Social workers deconstruct and reconstruct the way in which they implement and undertake their profession; also evident in the underlying notions of Pacific social work.

Social work as a contemporary profession in the Pacific

The recently revised *Global Definition of Social Work* put together by the International Association of Social Workers (IASSW) and the International Federation of Social Workers (IFSW) released in 2014 reads:

> Social Work is a practice-based profession and an academic discipline that promotes change and development, social cohesion, and the empowerment and liberation of people. Principles of social justice, human rights, collective responsibility and respect for diversities are central to social work. Underpinned by theories of social work, social sciences, humanities and indigenous knowledge, social work engages people and structures to address life challenges and enhance wellbeing. The above definition may be amplified at a national and/or regional levels.
>
> *(International Federation of Social Workers, 2018)*

Before this revised definition was established, there was a lack of inclusion and acknowledgement of indigenous practices or perspectives. The presence of *indigenous knowledge* is then of a major importance to not just social work as a profession, but to the way in which societal responses are developed and formed for local and regional communities. In essence, this addition also provides scope for western knowledges/dominant discourses to not be seen as the only way of thinking in social work, but to be challenged and complemented with diverse perspectives. The ability to also "amplify" this component across the broader global definition of social work is an encouraging step to the need to transform social work within a Pacific framing.

It is with this notion in mind that the final chapter of our book on Pacific social work anticipates to further explore the importance of having a shared platform to operate from, within and across when it comes to developing and implementing a profession as diverse as social work. In our attempt to effectively describe the underpinning of Pacific social work across the last 19 chapters, we purposefully use the notion of Pacific social work as a broad term and a genuine expression to reflect a collective and collaborative approach that is premised on the desire to effectively engage individuals, families, groups, community and wider society. But how can the profession be effective if it doesn't have a strong foundation in which to operate? And more so, how can the Pacific region and its vast and rich cultures benefit from meaningful and useful development if we haven't first considered what we believe or stand for as a profession? Therefore, it is important that we as social workers who work across practice, policy, research and education are constantly mindful of creating a professional response that is aligned to Pacific perspectives; ways of knowing, doing, being and becoming. At the same time, we are challenged by the resources, or the lack thereof, to provide interventions that may create sustainable changes due to the lack of political will, societal structures, systems or understandings of the true needs within the communities in which we operate and serve.

It is then our belief that the shared relationship that can occur between indigenous knowledge and its influence on social work as a profession globally can be used as this strong foundation to operate. Bringing the global down into the Pacific is also part of this approach; where we should be both mindful of social work as a global profession having an influence on what we do locally and regionally, but at the same time, there should be a reciprocal relationship occurring. Rather than believing that the global, including economic and political forces, should only determine what we do as social workers in the local and regional, we should also influence the global understanding of social work through our proactive approach to the local and regional. Pacific social work should then have a place at the global social work table, and even further support the development of social work practices across Oceania including Australia and New Zealand, Asia and beyond. Voices from the Pacific on social work and its various forms have not been traditionally discussed, heard or written about, hence the need for this book. At the same time, the need to ensure we can use our collective and shared experiences to articulate and voice our opinion on the world stage is also of importance. This means having a strong and determined outlook on the way in which we position Pacific social work as a valued and valid contribution to social work globally.

Indigeneity across the Pacific

The *Declaration of the Right of Indigenous Peoples* ratified by the United Nations on September 13, 2007 provides a global platform in which First Nations people can be understood, and treated in accordance with indigenous perspectives, places and spaces. Across the 46 Articles that make up the Declaration, key phrases are utilised to further position and make acknowledgement of Indigenous cultures; including the need to respect, empower and promote rights amongst societies where Indigenous people have been previously undermined or devalued. This includes article 23, which reads:

> Indigenous peoples have the right to determine and develop priorities and strategies for exercising their right to development. In particular, indigenous peoples have the right to be actively involved in developing and determining health, housing and other economic and social programmes affecting them and, as far as possible, to administer such programs through their own institutions.
>
> *(United Nations Declaration, 2008)*

As social workers, it is then imperative to position the notion of Pacific social work within this framing, with a view that such approaches to upholding Indigenous rights in and across the work we do is front and centre. However, this can be made harder when certain social systems, and its accompanying structure, continue to perpetuate the cycle of marginality Indigenous communities still continue to experience. The need to ensure that democratically elective governments are using their respective political will to promote this deceleration is also a telling tale when Indigenous people are still not provided the opportunity to be included and are grossly overrepresented across significant welfare, legal, health and social issues. Notwithstanding the Declaration being legally non-binding, 144 states supported the adoption of such rights – with 4 votes against and 11 abstentions, with a further 35 countries absent from voting. Of the 4 votes against, all are countries that have perpetuated gross atrocities against its First Nations and continue to thrive off Indigenous lands – Australia, Canada, New Zealand and the United States of America, but have since accepted and support the declaration. Of the 11 countries abstaining to vote, Samoa was one of them, and of the 35 absent counties, 10 were Pacific Island countries. In essence, this lack of buy in from our own Oceania region doesn't strike a level of confidence that governance structures, still to this day, are openly willing to uphold the various articles within the Deceleration.

Despite this lack of buy in, there is a ground swell towards indigeneity occurring across our Pacific region; notably through the humanitarian and development sector including social work (Mafile'o & Vakalahi, 2016; Ravulo, 2016). With many voices now starting to be heard more readily across the Islands and the diaspora community more broadly, the notion of Indigenous rights and the need to uphold such practices and its respective approaches is evolving. Slowly but surely, this movement is striving to question the status quo of existing societal structures, and why the heavy influence of capitalism and its relationship with materialism and individualism is being privileged over traditional Indigenous knowledge. Rather than position such discourse as being only for those from an Indigenous background to be involved in, the notion to decolonise western dominance over such peoples is being promoted as a shared approach and should include everyone. This means not just relegating Indigenous matters to Indigenous peoples alone, but to also educate and transform others around them to also be proactively involved in supporting such Indigenous knowledge and practices.

Social workers can be proactive in promoting practice, policy and research approaches that enable Indigenous Pacific people to see their indigeneity as a strength, an asset, and even a commodity that can better inform wider conversations around development (Rowe, Baldry & Earles, 2015). This notion of development, whether it be across an economic, financial, social or community context, can be underpinned by indigenous ways of knowing and doing (epistemology), and being and becoming (ontology) that can have a positive effect on not just their own communities but others. For example, across many indigenous Pacific cultures, the notion of collectivism is an important part of an individual identity; which then transforms the way in which families and communities operate. Rather than thinking that my own individual desire and aspirations are important to self alone, the collectivist perspective is on acknowledging that my goals and aspirations should be informed, shaped, moulded and carved in the context of other people including my immediate and extended family, kinship ties and fellow village and community members. This notion is further underpinned with the ideology that we all have a part to play in our families and communities and that our identities are reassured and fused into a bigger purpose of being part of the greater collective. Now imagine if this way of thinking was then incorporated into more capitalist, materialistic and individualistic societies. This is just one very basic example of how Indigenous perspective can be used to possibly shape the way in which we view ourselves, our families, our communities and societies. At the same time, we need to constantly challenge and disrupt western views who see this approach as archaic, old and not compatible with a modern way of thinking. Such limited views can continue to perpetuate the lessening of Indigenous perspectives. Instead, we should value such practices as a positive influence in modern society, in turn promoting positive development and wellbeing across the Pacific.

Paternalism in the Pacific and its diaspora

As social workers, we carry a level of power and control throughout the work we do. Many come into the profession with good intentions to make a difference, premising their desire to do so via a social justice lens. However, the various roles we are employed within do come with a position of influence; irrespective of whether it is across a small non-government agency or a large statutory setting. This is due to the way in which we as social workers may influence the outcomes associated with our own interaction with people across the many facets of the work we do. We engage with clients with the hope we can assist, but this also comes with an expectation that the people we are working with are also willing to receive the support we are offering; and if they aren't, this may then shape our interaction and ability to work effectively in achieving a particular desired outcome. And it is within this conundrum that our power as social workers can occur; we then determine whether people in contact with us do receive an outcome or not. Yes, it does require willingness on those we work with to be proactive in making progress to change, however, we generally can provide that bridge to become proactive for them to access the resources to do so, and at other times we may perpetuate the divide or lack of ability to effectively engage through our own views on the clients themselves. That is, we still operate with a level of expectation, hoping that the client will come on board with what we expect them to do. And it is within this notion that many Indigenous communities across Oceania are positioned. This paternalistic view continues to pervade funding committed by foreign entities like Australia and New Zealand to the region; with expectations that such funding is provided to support development in a manner that produces certain results. At the same time, these expectations may also create an ongoing level of dependency on foreign aid, which in turn perpetuates the perception of the Island states and territories being the poorer cousins of the other larger economies in the region. Such ideologies can then further discount the need to utilise Indigenous knowledge, perspectives and practices in areas of development, as we perceive the ability for the larger countries to provide aid as an indication that west is best, white is right; again at the sacrifice of traditional approaches. This tension should be acknowledged in Pacific social work practice, policy and research, with a view to ensure the relationship with Indigenous cultures is not seen as the lesser of the two. Instead, an intention to collaborate between the social work profession, and the people it is interacting with, is imperative in assuring the negative effects of paternalism is counteracted.

Therefore, we need to work within this tension – seeing this as part and parcel of trying to effectively navigate Pacific social work and its application across the region, and with the diaspora community in which we are serving. Even in the larger countries our communities reside, like Australia, New Zealand, USA and Europe, the need to ensure cultural perspectives are included in the work we do is vital. It can be easier to employ dominant perspectives that underpin social work in such westernised settings, where the individual is seen as the key focus at the detriment of then not understanding the bigger and wider connection to family and community. However, time and time again, such approaches may not fully engage the individual adequately in their many contexts, which in turn creates further issues across their psycho-social wellbeing. Instead, by utilising a social work approach like anti-oppressive or anti-discriminatory, we not only strive to acknowledge and address the structural issues that perpetuate such social and welfare concerns, we also strive to challenge and create sustainable options for positive change and inclusion.

Deconstructing and reconstructing social work across Pacific spaces

Pacific social work with its emphasis to truly understand the Pacific context and spaces in which Pacific people exist, should be further nuanced and shaded with expectations that are shared in nature, rather than applied based on existing professional rhetoric and expectations. The need to ensure Pacific epistemologies and ontologies feature heavily in the practices, policy and research undertaken with Pacific communities is not static or fixed, which is often the same across human societies and cultures globally. Even Indigenous ways on knowing, doing, being and becoming evolve in their countries of origin, and it's important that social workers are also aware of such change. Traditional practices and approaches that may be esteemed by one generation may be implemented, but can also be reshaped and reformed across different settings. For example, in village life, certain traditional practices may be more evident and practiced in that particular setting or context, and esteemed as being more valued and desired. Such practices may still occur in peri-urban and city dwellings, but other factors are also at play like the need to keep up with capitalistic commitments outside the village, for example, financial needs associated with accommodation, transportation, educational and employment commitments beyond the traditional roles undertaken in the family. It is within this ever-changing landscape that Pacific people have also learnt to adapt, continuously learning new ways of knowing and doing, being and becoming whilst also balancing their strong commitment to traditional ways. Hence, as social workers striving to implement notions of Pacific social work, we are needing to constantly deconstruct and reconstruct the way in which we work with individuals, families and communities across practice, policy and research. Rather than thinking our approach is linear, it is more characterised by the peaks and troughs of the land and sea in which we navigate. It is within this visual metaphor that the following perspective has been developed to further highlight the way in which Pacific social work may occur, and how we as practitioners need to truly understand our own contribution to ensuring Pacific communities are able to successfully navigate their own space and place.

Within this metaphor lies the need to promote an ongoing commitment to be a reflexive social worker, focused on being critical in the way in which one operates as a practitioner. The profession is underpinned by the need to be mindful of how one positions themselves through their own personal and professional lenses; and it is then within this space that social workers should exist. That is, the need to be consistently and consciously aware of how social work perspectives utilised in working with Pacific communities should be deconstructed and examined to understand its impact; whilst also reconstructing approaches with Indigenous knowledges to the betterment of the working being undertaken. It is hoped that through this approach, a more meaningful relationship occurs between social work as a profession and the ability to truly collaborate with the Pacific people we come into contact through this role.

> Visualise the movement of waves on the shoreline of a beach, where the water meets the land. As the wave comes into contact with the sand, the sand is then picked up by the wave, and the water then moves back out to sea, but is now transporting part of the land with it. As the waves continue to come into contact with the shoreline, both the water and the land is transformed through such motion. However, there is a reciprocal relationship between the waves of the sea and the land, where their connection and relationship are both meaningfully informed by each other. The wave is deconstructed and transformed as a flatter flow of water over the sand but is then reconstructed as it is then brought back into the ocean in which it exists.
>
> It is within this relationship between the wave from the sea and the sand from the land in which we see Pacific social work occurring. The wave represents the existing body of knowledge we use as social workers, which may be informed by western perspectives and practices. As it meets with the shoreline, which represents Indigenous knowledge, certain elements of this interaction are picked up, and taken with it as it moves back out into the wider field of practice as a reconstruction of its former shape. This body of water is then positively influenced by its interaction with the shoreline; the various Indigenous ways of knowing, doing, being and becoming, that its reformation as a wave is meaningfully informed, with a view that when it comes back into contact with the shoreline, it continues to deconstruct and reconstruct accordingly.

Conclusion

Throughout the chapter, an emphasis to be inclusive of Indigenous knowledges and its practices have been given with a view that this should be a shared space in social work. It is important that we end this piece by further reiterating this message – that achieving an engaging and meaningful approach in and across Pacific social work is one where everyone is involved. This means non-Pacific and Pacific people co-creating, co-designing, co-shaping and co-existing across the way in which social work is undertaken within its many shapes and forms. It is within this context that true decoloniality can occur and everyone is able to share a common goal in promoting common unity. And when placed together, this common unity can effectively shape a more responsive and robust community, poised to be more inclusive. Even though social work as a profession can be at the forefront of achieving this across the region through practice, policy and research, the aspiration to also work collaboratively with other professions including psychology, law and medicine; including traditional, visual and performing arts, economics and politics, should occur. Through this, we can optimistically strive to accomplish the greater outcome of fostering societal expectations that genuinely uphold and implement UN Declarations, foreign aid, democratically elected governance structures and community strategies that make a difference.

REFLECTIVE QUESTIONS

1. Social work in the Pacific is not for the faint hearted – or else we simply tow the systems line. It is an exciting space to be in, but a challenging one as well. What are some of these possible challenges? How could such challenges be counteracted?
2. The inclusion of the word indigenous in the IFSW's global definition of social work is a part of the ongoing battle at a worldwide level for recognition of indigenous communities; and to that extent the Pacific could play a critical role in this space if they looked to themselves in the first instance, looked at context to develop their own models to drive their own research and policy. What are some of these Pacific perspectives that could aid in Pacific social work?
3. Understanding how we develop our own professional perspectives from our own personal views; including biases is important. How can we effectively ensure we are consistently inclusive of indigenous knowledges in social work practice, policy and research?

References

International Federation of Social Workers. (2018). *Global definition of social work*. Retrieved from www.ifsw.org/what-is-social-work/global-definition-of-social-work/

Mafile'o, T. & Vakalahi, H. F. O. (2016). Indigenous social work across borders: Expanding social work in the South Pacific. *International Social Work*, 61(4). https://doi.org/10.1177/0020872816641750

Ravulo, J. (2016). Pacific epistemologies in professional social work practice, policy and research. *Asia Pacific Journal of Social Work and Development*, 26(4), 191–202. https://doi.org/10.1080/02185385.2016.1234970

Rowe, S., Baldry, E. & Earles, W. (2015). Decolonising social work research: Learning from critical indigenous approaches. *Australian Social Work*, *68*(3), 296–308. Retrieved from www.tandfonline.com/doi/pdf/10.1080/0312407X.2015.1024264?needAccess =true

United Nations Declaration. (2008). United Nations Declaration on the Rights of Indigenous Peoples. *United Nations General Assembly*, (Resolution 61/295), 10. https://doi.org/10.1093/iclqaj/24.3.577

Suggested further readings/websites

Seminal piece on the inclusion of Pacific perspectives in social work theory; including the notion *the wave framework* as a means to include diverse perspectives: Mafile'o, T. (2001). Pasifika social work theory. *Social Work Review*, (Spring), 10–13.

Social Work Regional Resource Centre of Oceania (SWRROC) is a new initiative supported by the International Association of Schools of Social Work (IASSW). As per their very active Facebook page, they are "a network of Pacific social work educators and practitioners collaborating to advance Pacific social work practice, policy, research and education to benefit Pacific peoples' social development": www.facebook.com/pacificsocialwork

INDEX

Page numbers in *italics* refer to figures. Page numbers in **bold** refer to tables.

2030 Sustainable Development Agenda 199

abortion 131
acculturation/acculturative stress 144–145
adaptability 62
adult offenders 90–99
Affirming Works (AW) 74
aga-i-fanua (rule of the land) 12–15, 20
Agenda 21 60
aiga (family) 13, 16, 18–19
Akono'anga Māori 27–28
alcohol use 139–147
Alefaio, S. 74
Alexeyeff, K. 166
Altman, D. 167
Alzheimer's disease 153
American Geriatrics Society 153
Anae, M. 87
anti-oppressive approach 48–49, 92, 96, **96**
anti-social behaviour 92
Appel, J. 215
Archibald, J. 31
Auckland Institute of Technology (AUT) 111
Australia Pacific Technical College (APTC) 111

Baba, T. 189
Bainimarama, F. 163
Barreneche, G. 16
Belsky, J. 173

Berry, J. W. 144
Betel nut 141
binge-drinking of kava 142
bio-psycho-social approach 48–49
"blackbirding" era 6
"Blue Pacific" identity 199
bottom-up developments 106–107
Bull, S. 94
Bywater, J. 135

Carteret islanders 63–64
case management 96–97
case studies: on adult offenders 97–98; *aga-i-fanua* and 13–14; on child protection 121–122; on data collection 168; on elders 157; on family and domestic violence 176–178; on kava consumption 143–145; on mental health 53–55; on natural disasters 69–77; on same-sex relationships 163–164; on youth offending 85–86
Case Studies on Climate and Disaster Resilient Development in the Pacific 61
Chanwai, G. 143–144
child abuse and neglect *see* family and domestic violence
child protection 121–122
China: influence of 5
Christianity 130, 167
civil society organisations (CSOs) 201–203
climate change 6, 58–65, **59**, 68

Coady, N. 24, 26
Coalition of Rainforest Nations (CfRN) 60
cognitive behaviour therapy (CBT) 140
collectivism 226
colonisation 189–190, 198, 210
Coming of Age in Samoa (Mead) 167
Committee against Violence against Women (CAVAW) 180
communal lifestyles 16–19, 23
Community Based Organisations (CBOs) 202
Community Café 74, 76
community development 102–112
Community Development Learning Centres 109
Community-Led Millennium Development Goal Acceleration Pilot Project (CLMAP) 111
community organising 50
community ownership 107
community resilience 73–74, 78
community-village resilience 68–78
Comparison of Pacific, Māori, and European Violent Youth Offenders in New Zealand, A 81
Convention on the Elimination of All Forms of Discrimination Against Women (CEDAW) 117
Convention on the Rights of the Child (CRC) 117
Conventions on the Rights of Persons with Disabilities (CRPD) 38–41, 43–44
Cook Islands 26–28
Corporate Plan of the Department of Environment 60
Council of Regional Organisations of the Pacific (CROP) 40, 200–201, 204
criminogenic factors 93
crisis/task-centred approach 140
critical reflection: poem on 135–136
CSO Engagement Strategy 201
cultural divide 17
Cultural-Elder Advisors of SUNGO 69–70
culturally appropriate approaches 90–99
Cyclone Gita 69, 74–77

data collection 168, 201, 210, 212, 217
Declaration of the Right of Indigenous Peoples 225
decolonisation/decoloniality 6, 9, 23, 29, 210, 214–217, 230
Deeper Silence, A (Spratt) 39

dementia 153
Deportation of Non-Citizen Criminals scheme 95
deportation policy 95–96
Developing and Implementing a Case Management Model for Young People with Complex Needs 87
disability 37–44
disaster response 68–77, 72
District Development Authorities 109
Dove 63
drug use 139–147
Durie, M. 185, 189–190
duty of care 27–28

Ebacher, C. 16
ecological systems theory (EST) 24, 80, 118, 152
education, social work 156–157
Efi, T. A. T. T. T. 13, 30, 69–70, 119
elders 150–158
empowerment 108, 110–111
Endemann-Pulotu, K. 118
engagement 120
environmental justice 58–65
environmental social work 64–65
epistemology 12–16
equality 199
Erickson, E. 151

fa'aaloalo (respect) 12, 14, 16–17
fa'afafine 162, 167–169
Fa'afaletui approach 213
fa'a Samoa 202
fa'asinomaga 70
fahu 115
Falelolo, M. M. 143
family and domestic violence 26, 81, 172–181, 202
Family and Traditional Child Protection System model 179
Family Protection Act (Vanuatu) 175
Family Protection Bill (Solomon Islands) 175
family-reliance 69
family systems approach 52
family-tree approach 105
Farrelly, T. 86, 216
Fehoko, E. 142
feminist theory 174
figurative language 30
Filer, C. 63
Fonofale 24, 54, 86–87, 118–119
food security 6

foreign aid 5
Forster 175
Framework for Pacific Regionalism 199, 204
Fua, C. 143
future directions 223–230

Galuega toe Fuata'ina 69–70
gender equality 61, 117, 173–174, 201–204
genograms 52
Global Definition of Social Work 223–224
"global gay identity" 167
global migration and resettlement 184–191
Global Sustainable Development Goals 111–112
Grattan, F. J. 19
group work 97

harm minimisation 145
hate crimes 167–168
Hau'ofa, E. 5
Hayes, H. 94
Helu, F. 142
Herdt, G. 164
homophobic violence 167–168
Ho'okele model 151–152
Ho'oponopono 24
Huffer, E. 17
human rights 6, 108, 110

identity: labels of 6–7, **7**
Ife, J. 103, 108
images 29–30
incarceration rates 80–81, 93
Incheon Strategy 40
indigeneity 199, 225–226
Indigenous frameworks 105–106, 155–156
Indigenous rights 225–226
Information and Knowledge Management for Climate Change (IKM4CC) Strategic Framework 59–60
Integrated Community Development Policy 109
International Association of Community Development (IACD) 103–104
International Association of Schools of Social Work (IASSW) 59, 128, 223
international development assistance 5
International Federation of Social Workers (IFSW) 128, 223
International Lesbian, Gay, Bisexual, Trans and Intersex Association 161
intimate partner violence *see* family and domestic violence
Ioane, J. 81

Johnston, D. 74
Joint Centre for Disaster Research (JCDR) 74
Jones, R. 135
Jorgensen, D. 63

Kahn, M. W. 143
kainga (family) 12
Kakala framework 211–212
Kamu, L. 19
Karlan, D. S. 215
Kato Fetu: Review of the Pacific Mental Health and Addiction Research Agenda 49
kava: alcohol and drug consumption 139–147
Kay, A. 105
kinship systems 23, 202
Knauft, B. 165

laelae 166
Lalaga Model 18
Lambie, I. 81
landownership 63–64
Le Va 49–50
LGBTQI+ 161–170, **169**

Macanawai, S. 43
MacPherson, C. 17
MacPherson, L. 17
Madraiwiwi, J. 189, 198
Mafile'o, T. 12, 104–105
mahi tahi 107
Malinowski, B. 164
Mana Moana 28–31
Mango Tree 42–43
Māori 84, 86–87, 93–94
marijuana/cannabis 141, 143
matai (chief) 15–16, 19, 98
Mataira, P. 214
Maxwell, G. 94, 96
Mead, M. 167
Melanesia 63–64
Melanesian Spearhead Group 4–5
mental health and wellbeing 47–56, 153
Mental Health Week 51
Meo-Sewabu, L. 198, 212
metaphors 30
Micronesian Presidents' Group 4–5
migration 154, 184–191
Millennium Development Goals (MDGs) 60, 197
Mooney, H. 86
Morelli, P. 214
motivational interviewing 140

236 Index

Mulitalo-Lauta, P. T. 18
multidisciplinary approach 86–87
Munford, R. 104–105

Nabobo-Baba, U. 86, 106, 188–189, 212, 216
Nai Dabedabe 42–43
Nakhid, C. 81
narrative approach 140
narratives 31
National Climate Change Policy Framework (Fiji) 60
National Climate Compatible Development Management Policy (Papua New Guinea) 60–61
natural disasters 6, 68–78
Naylor, B. 94
ngakau aro'a 28
Nga Vaka o Kainga Tapu 174
NIUPacH (New Indigenous Unity of Pacific Humanitarians) 75
non-communicable diseases 6
non-heteronormativity 161–170
Nosa, V. 142
No teia tuatau 28

Ofanoa, M. 142
offending trends 80–82
Open Worksheet 146
Oxfam 76–77

Pacific Community 50–51, 104
Pacific Conceptual Framework 155
Pacific Conference of Churches (PCC) 5
Pacific Disability Forum 38, 40
Pacific Framework for the Rights of Persons with Disabilities (PFRPD) 40–41, 44
Pacific geo-politics 4–8
Pacific Identity and Wellbeing Scale 210
Pacific-Indigenous theories and models 22–32, *25*
Pacific Islands Association of Non-Government Organisation (PIANGO) 5
Pacific Islands Development Forum 5
Pacific Islands Forum (PIF) 5, 198
Pacific Islands Framework for Action on Climate Change 2006–2015 60
Pacific Platform for Action (PPA) on the Advancement of Women and Gender Equality 203–204
Pacific Platform for Action on Gender Equality and Women's Human Rights 2018–2030 198, 202–204

Pacific Regional Framework 117
Pacific social work: community development and 102–112; community-village resilience and 68–78; culturally appropriate approaches and 90–99; defining 4; disability and 37–44; elders and 150–158; environmental justice and 58–65; family and domestic violence and 172–181; future directions for 223–230; global migration and resettlement and 184–191; introduction to 3–9; kava, alcohol and drug consumption and 139–147; mental health and wellbeing and 47–56; research paradigm for 209–218; sexual and gender diversity and 161–170; sexual and reproductive health and wellbeing and 125–136; social policy processes and 197–204; theories and models for 22–32; values and beliefs and 11–20; women and children and 114–122; youth justice and 79–88
Pacific Theological College (PTC) 5
Pākehā 81
Pan American Health Organisation (PAHO) 127
Papua New Guinea (PNG) 60–61, 63–64, 109
participation: full 199
participatory cultural approaches 61
paternalism 227–228
Patterson, A. C. 186
Pearce, J. 105
Percival, T. 81
personal as political 108
piri'anga 27–28
policy organisations **134**
Polynesian Leaders' Group 4–5
positionality 215–217
Powaseu, I. 43
Power, R. 143
Presterudstuen, G. H. 167
principles of practice for community development 105–109
process-oriented approach 108–109
protective factors: for family and domestic violence 179–180; for youth offending 82, **83–84**
proverbs 30–31, 114–116
psychosocial development: stages of 151
Pulotu-Endemann, F. K. 87, 118
Putnam, R. D. 186

Qalo, R. 17
qauri 162, 165, 167

racism 6
Ramos-Flores, H. 16
rational choice theory 90–91
Ratuva, S. 189
Ravulo, J. 82, 146
reciprocity 118, 187
relocation 61–64
research paradigm: Pacific-Indigenous 209–218, **213**
resettlement 184–191
resilience 62, 68–78
respect 119
restorative justice 94, 96, **96**
rights-based approach 41, 44
risk factors for youth offending 82, **83–84**
ritualised homosexuality 164–165
Roffee, J. 94
Rotuivaqali, M. T. 189

Saili Matagi 98
Sam, D. L. 144
same-sex relationships 161–170
Samoan perspectives/culture 12–20, **20**
Sanga, K. 107
Schmich, L. 143
Schmidt, J. 167
Scott, G. 82
Secretariat of Pacific Community (SPC) 5, 50–51, 200, 203
Secretariat of the Pacific Regional Environment Program (SPREP) 60
self-help approach 110
self-reliance 69
Sentencing Act (2002) 97
service learning 16, 20
sexual and gender diversity 161–170
sexual and reproductive health and wellbeing 125–136, **128**
sexuality: definition of 127
sexual violence 130–131
Siegel, S. 144
Small Island Developing States (SIDS) global agenda 199
social capital 80, 186; change 109; exclusion 81; justice 108, 110; policy implementation 201–202; policy processes 197–204, *200*; protection 6, 189
solesolevaki tradition 107, 187
South Pacific Association of Theological Schools (SPATS) 5
space: vacating 115
Spoonley, P. 185
strengths-based approach (SBA) 120

Strengths Enhancing Evaluation Research (SEER) 210, 214–215
structural violence 91–92, 96
substance use 139–147
Sustainable Development Goals (SDG) 40, 51, 60, 197

Tā'anga'anga'ia 28
talanoa 4, 9, 15, 42, 51–52, 54–55, 76–77, 86, 97–98, 212, 216–217
Talanoa HUBBS 75, *75*, 77, 77
Task Centred Model 24
Taufe'ulungaki, A. 120
tautua (service) 15–16
terminology 6–8, **7**, 162, **169**, **191**
Te Whanau Awhina model 94
Te Whare Tapa Wha 24
Thaman, K. H. 211
"third gender" 165–166
Tikotikoca, Leslie 40–41
tobacco 141–142
tomboys 169
Tonga 51, 60, 69, 74–77
transnationalism 185–187
Tulele Peisa 63–64
Tupu'anga Coffee/Café 74–77
turanga 27–28
Turanga Māori 26–28

United Nations Children's Fund (UNICEF) 173, 179–180
United Nations Development Program (UNDP) 104, 111
United Nations Economic and Social Council 5
United Nations Permanent Forum on Indigenous Issues 188
University of the South Pacific (USP) 40, 111
Uo, R. 131–132
Urville, J. D. d' 4

Vā 49–52, 114–122
va fealoaloa'i (respectful relationship) 14, 16–17
Vaioleti, T. 86
Vaka, S. 212
values and beliefs 11–20
Vanua (land) 43, 186–190, 212
Vanuatu 60–61
Vanuatu Mental Health Policy and Strategic Plan 50
vasu 115
Veenstra, G. 186
veitokoni 118

veiwekani 202
Vertovec, S. 185–186
Village Collective (VC) 132
vision 105
vulnerability 61–62, 68–78

wā 117
Walsh-Tapiata, W. 105, 198
wantok system 108, 202
Ward, C. 144
wellbeing: concept of 126; continuum of 26; defining 188–189; indicators of 190; measures of 210; sexual 127

Whitehead, J. 94
women and children 114–122; *see also* family and domestic violence
Women's Centre (Vanuatu) 180
words: power of 29
World Health Organization (WHO) 117, 127, 130, 153
World Report on Disability 38

Yellow Ribbon programme 98
youth justice 79–88
youth offending 79–88, 93
youth unemployment 6